“Beautifully Unbroken”

A Life-Changing Invention: Born of Loss, Cancer, Courage, and Faith.

LISA F. CRITES

Printed in the United States of America

First Printing Edition, 2026

I S B N 979-8-99031285-2 (Ebook)

I S B N 979-8-9903128-6-9 (Paperback)

I S B N 978-1-99704029-3 (Hardcover)

Copyright Case ID: 1-15188469311

Dedication

This book is dedicated to the memory of two of my childhood friends, Lee Anne Swinger and Shawna Lane Godwin, both taken far too soon by aggressive forms of breast cancer.

I would also like to acknowledge Dr. Emran Imami. Not only for his friendship and clinical expertise, but for helping make me "whole" again after the severe complications I experienced from breast cancer.

I also dedicate this book to the memory of my mother, whose care, guidance, loyalty, love, and strong Christian faith shaped my life. I would not be the person I am today without her.

I would also like to thank Amazon Publication Studio for their advocacy in bringing this project to life, and the Historic Cocoa Village Playhouse for oversight and support in recording the audiobook.

Disclaimer

Beautifully Unbroken is a memoir based on the personal experiences of the author, Lisa Faye Crites. The content of this book is intended for educational and inspirational purposes only and should not be considered a substitute for professional medical, legal, or financial advice. Readers are encouraged to consult qualified professionals regarding any health, business, or personal decisions.

Authors Note

Thank you for reading *Beautifully Unbroken*. My hope is that this book brings encouragement to breast cancer patients who are searching for hope, that it motivates inventors who need that PUSH (Push Until Something Happens), and demonstrates to anyone who needs reassurance that faith and inspiration come from above — you simply must ask.

I also hope my story serves as a reminder that there is always light after darkness, but sometimes you must search for it. There is always sunshine after the pouring rain, though at times we must first endure the storm. Prepare as if tomorrow is the first day of the rest of your life – for the opportunity to live with courage, authenticity, resilience, gratitude, and originality -CARGO.

Let us also remember the hundreds of thousands of breast cancer patients who fought this storm and survived, along with those who fought this disease with grace and fortitude but ultimately lost the battle.

And finally, I genuinely believe laughter through tears is one of life's most powerful and healing emotions.

Contents

CHAPTER 1
The Voice That Shaped My Life

If I had to pinpoint the one thing that has carried me through every twist and turn of my life, it would be my voice. Not just the strong, deep sound that comes out when I speak, but the drive, the curiosity, the insistence to be heard and to listen. That voice has been my compass, my anchor, and my weapon long before television journalism, inventions, or adult responsibilities came into play.

Let me properly introduce myself. My name is Lisa Crites. I'm an American journalist, a patented inventor, a medical magazine columnist, and now an author. But before any of those titles came to fruition — before the bright studio lights and tight deadlines — I always had a yearning to understand the world. That hunger to chase the truth, to uncover stories that mattered, shaped everything I became.

My professional career took off in the chaotic and adrenaline-fueled world of health and medical reporting. Wires, mics, directors speaking in your ear during live shots, scripts handed over at the last second, and that relentless tick-tock of deadlines that never stopped. I reported and anchored for Central Florida News 13, a 24-hour news station, and previously a CNN affiliate in Orlando. I then worked with America's Health Network, taping on the backlot of Universal

Studios, which ultimately became the Discovery Health Network.

I also worked with WCPX-TV Channel 6 in Orlando, (now WKMG), WSIL News 3 in Harrisburg, Illinois, and their bureau, KPOB Channel 15, Poplar Bluff, Missouri; Hometown Health, PBS, and the Travel Channel. Each assignment carved me sharper, taught me to stay calm under pressure, ask the questions that mattered, and most importantly, find the human-interest narrative buried inside every headline. Eventually, I moved behind the scenes as a media strategist, then news consultant for Gannett News Service, teaching print journalists how to use their voices, speak on camera, and become television reporters. That consulting role reminded me how powerful the gift of voice truly was.

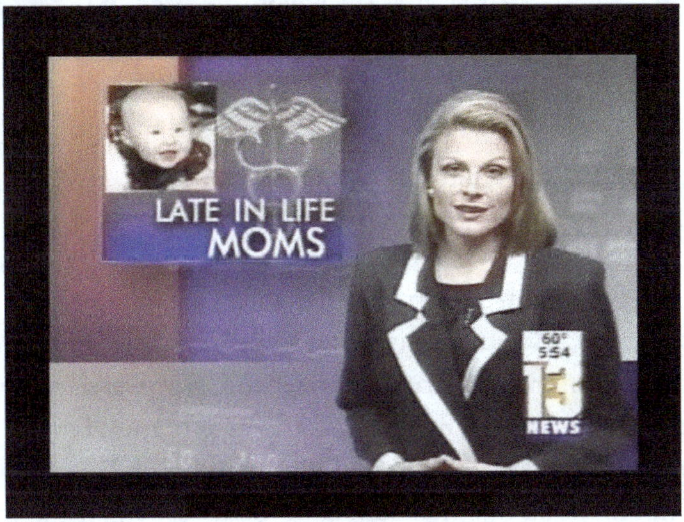

Working in the Channel 13 Studios in Orlando

Medical journalism has carried me through a 30-year career. The news field took me from reporting to anchoring, to media strategy in the corporate offices of two large hospital systems; from covering the Natalee Holloway missing persons search in Aruba, to becoming a patented inventor of a medical device, ghostwriting guest columns and medical journals for doctors across the United States, and serving as a health and medical print columnist for a national magazine.

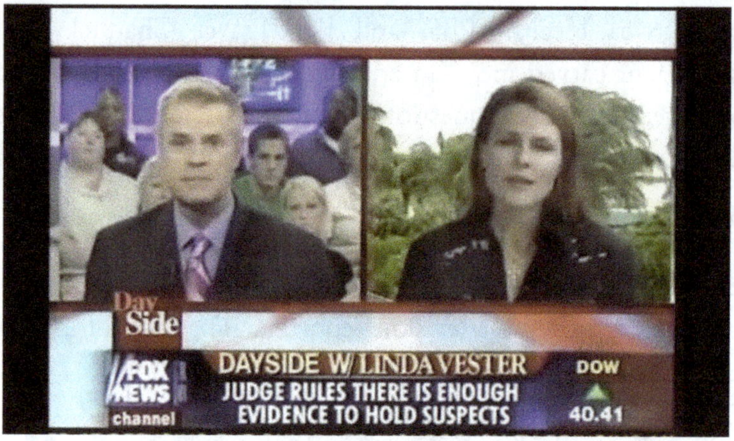

In Aruba reporting on FOX News

Long before the cameras and the accolades, my story began in a far quieter place: a family farm in Southeast Missouri, smack in the middle of the Midwest.

I am a true farmer's daughter, raised between the privilege of wide-open fields and the pressures of a stern, uncompromising father. On one hand, we were extremely fortunate. Ours was a home always open to friends, family, and animals. We were members of the country club and had a swimming pool, one that seemed to be used by half the town every summer. We had trampolines, several motorcycles, a pond behind the house where we could fish, and acres of land that felt endless to a child.

On the other hand, because my father was a farmer, our entire lives revolved around the weather. Every meal, every conversation, every mood depended on whether the crops would survive the season. He had an unbelievably strong work ethic, which made him an exceptional provider for me, my mother, and my three brothers. But he was also incredibly strict and no-nonsense, not easy to navigate as a little girl. I cried often; he had a way of saying things that cut right through me. I would hear my mother say quietly, *"Gary, you cannot speak to your daughter the same way you speak to your sons. She's more sensitive."*

Looking back now, at 59, I can understand some of his actions, but I still believe his rules went too far. My mother, who managed him well, would remind him, *"You have good children. When they make mistakes, you are irrational and too hard on them."* She was right. His reactions to even the smallest missteps were overwhelming. Growing up under a man like that was not easy, yet I also know he believed deeply in preparing my brothers and me for a life built on an uncompromising work ethic, Christian values, advanced education, and altruism.

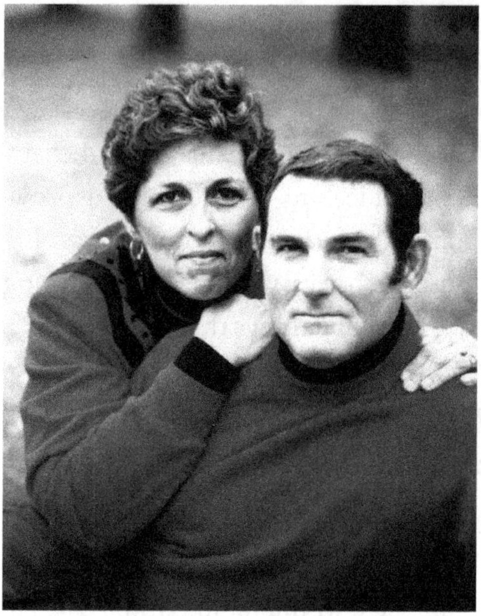

My Mother and Father (Gary and Dianne Crites)

My mother was our buffer. She stood between us and his intensity, softening the hard edges where she could. My two older brothers worked closely with my father on the farm, while my younger brother and I spent most of our time with her. Being her constant companion created a deep bond and made me her staunch protector. It also meant that as I grew older, more mature, and mentally stronger, my father and I clashed often. Some of those disagreements were generational, but others were simply about gender. He came from a world where women followed a narrow script of marriage and motherhood, a script I was never destined for. I was independent, ambitious, and determined to build a life that looked nothing like the one he had imagined for me back in the Midwest.

I watched the women in earlier generations of my family either have no financial independence or relinquish financial control entirely to their husbands, except for my paternal grandmother, who was elected Recorder of Deeds in the 1960s and held a significant political position in the county where I grew up. I also saw how my father controlled my mother's spending and decision-making, and I vowed early that I would never allow myself to be financially dependent on a man. I wanted autonomy, financially, emotionally, and intellectually. I made choices based on what was best for me, my journalism career, and my business goals. And while that strength has served me well, not every man has known what to do with a woman who didn't need him for her survival.

Growing up with three brothers, no sisters, and as the only granddaughter on my father's side shaped me profoundly. I was spoiled but being surrounded by boys, I learned early to think the way men think and, more importantly, to see men as friends first: allies, partners in crime. Maybe that's why I've always had lifelong platonic friendships with men. At the same time, being raised under a strict, iron-willed father gave me a kind of armor. My brothers were expected to be tough, but I'm not sure that same expectation was ever placed on me, which made it all the more striking when my father looked at me one day and said, *"Lisa, I raised you to be tough, but not this tough."* That strength, combined with a deeply ingrained independence, has been both my anchor and, admittedly, a complicating force in every personal relationship throughout my life.

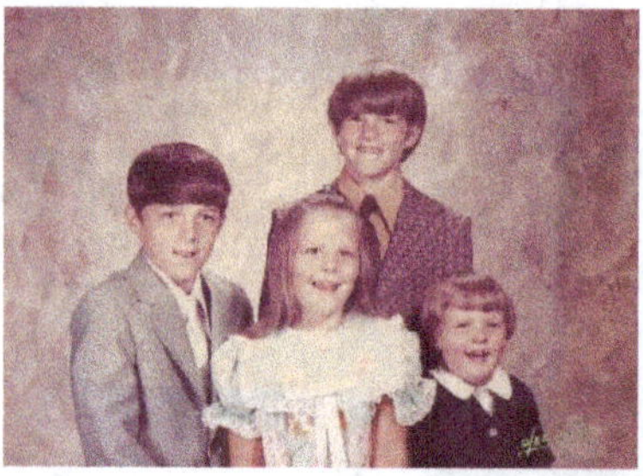

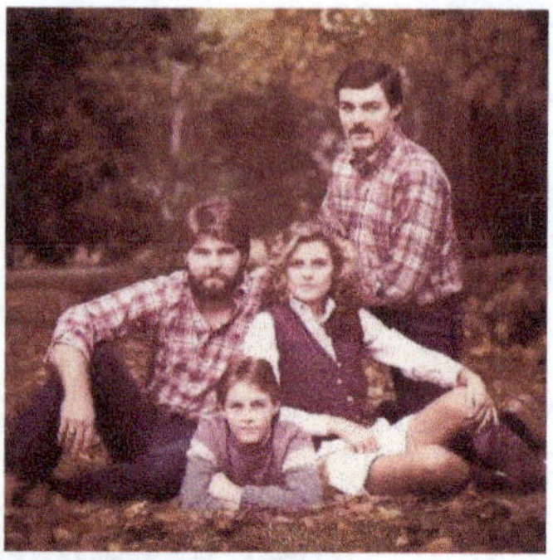

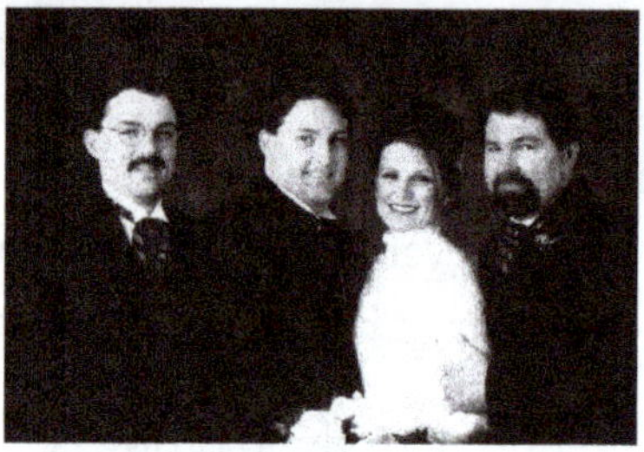

Me and My Brothers

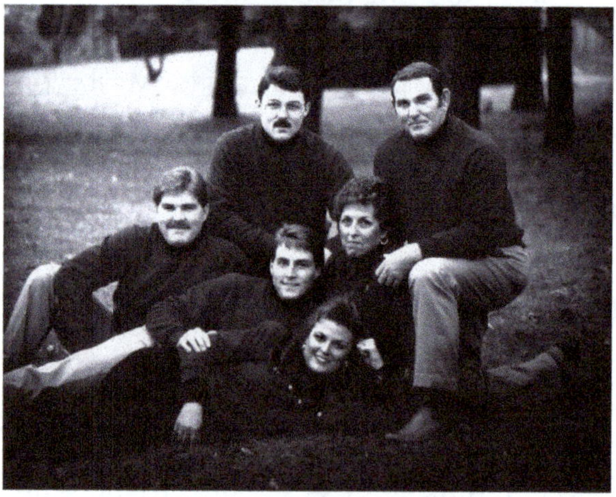

The Crites Family
(From left to right: My brothers: Shawn, Andy, Charles, Me, Mom and Dad)

Today, my father is 86 and struggles with a host of health issues: cardiac anomalies, kidney failure, yet remains externally strong as an ox, with a muscular build most men couldn't attain in their thirties or forties. When I look at him now, I can understand his soul in ways my younger self could not. That understanding has softened even the sharpest edges of my memory.

Our town, Essex, Missouri, had a population of barely 500, and life revolved around school, high school sports, church, family, friends, and the farmer's soil. Everyone knew everyone. Step out of line, and the town would know before you did. My mother would look at me and say, *"A little bird told me what you did."* She always knew. There was beauty in that closeness.

And then, of course, there are the childhood memories imprinted in you forever, the ones that just live inside you like small, unshakeable pieces of your heart. Many of mine are tied to Christmas at the family farmhouse. Every year, we would gather with my father's sister's family, the Millers, crowding around the piano beside the Christmas tree, singing carols, my father's beautiful, operatic voice outshining us all.

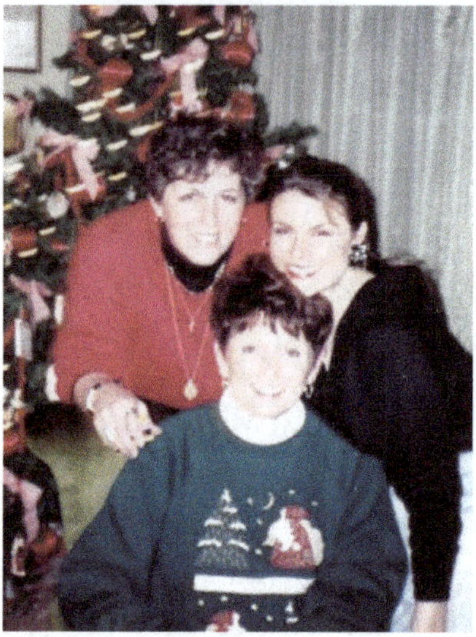

My Mother, Aunt Faye, and Me

The winter months also brought snowstorms that shut the town down entirely, and those days became some of my favorite memories. My father would haul one of his massive John Deere tractors out of the shed, hook up a giant sled, and suddenly half the town was on board. We'd slide across the snowy streets, forty people packed together, screaming and laughing as the tractor whipped around corners.

People would fly off, roll in the snow, and scramble back on. Doors stayed unlocked. Neighbors watched each other's children. That was the rhythm of my childhood: freedom and discipline, warmth and structure, laughter and fear, all stitched together into the red, white, and blue tapestry of small-town America.

Faith was the backbone of our world. My family was deeply Christian, and church was never optional. Every Sunday, we dressed up and went, no excuses, no skipping. Summers meant Bible school, and our social lives flowed seamlessly from the classroom into the pews. Christianity was woven into the rhythm of our days from the very beginning. I was sprinkled in the Methodist church as a baby and later baptized again in the Baptist church.

My mother was an avid reader who talked about Christian teachings constantly. She discussed theology, quoted Scripture, and genuinely loved learning about other religions. She kept a book titled *The Book of the Bible* and often spoke about religious beliefs from around the world. But her most consistent message was simple: hand your worries to God. Whenever I felt upset or unsure, which was often, she would hug me and say, *"Lisa, get down on your knees and pray. God will take care of this."* That mindset shaped the way I approached every challenge throughout my life. Because of my unusually strict and sheltered upbringing, college felt like stepping into a whole new world. I was never promiscuous; that was simply not my nature, but having real space to breathe, with genuine freedom, was a significant adjustment.

When you grow up in a town of a few hundred people, with a father on the school board and a mother who knows every family on every street, there is no room for mischief. College lifted that invisible weight. I attended Murray State University in Western Kentucky, just as all three of my brothers did. My father would joke that he practically owned a building on campus; he had children enrolled there from 1980 to 1995, and for seven of those years, two of us were there at the same time.

My path to journalism began unexpectedly. I had arrived at Murray State on a four-year scholarship as a classically trained pianist, set to study in the music department. But even as a freshman, I knew music was not my destiny. My heart was in storytelling. One day, I wandered up three flights of stairs to the journalism department, lingered in the newsroom, and stood there mesmerized, watching students draft stories and produce newscasts. By my sophomore year, I had switched my major to journalism, though I continued private classical piano lessons with my music professor through the end of my junior year. Murray State ran a working college newsroom that produced live newscasts covering local happenings, campus events, city council meetings, college sports, and community news. It was as close to the real thing as a student could get.

The last semester of my junior year brought an opportunity that would shape me enormously: a coveted internship at WSIL, the ABC affiliate in southern Illinois. It was my first experience in an authentic professional newsroom. I left campus for the semester, took classes at a local junior college, and spent my weekends working, half days during the week, full days on Saturday and Sunday. It was exhausting alongside my studies. My friends were back at Murray State enjoying Greek life, football games, and social events, while I was spending weekends writing stories about communities across multiple states. Most Midwest television stations cover vast territories, such as Illinois, Missouri, and Kentucky, so even as an intern at the Illinois ABC affiliate, I was filing news for the entire tri-state area.

Calloway County, Kentucky, where Murray State sat, was technically a dry county, though still one of the wettest dry counties in the state, thanks to the college. My sorority sisters and I would pile into a car and drive twenty minutes into Tennessee, a ritual we jokingly called *"Going South,"* to buy alcohol or hang out at a small bar called Jack's. It felt daring at the time, but looking back, it was harmless fun.

Greek life in the '80s was one of the most meaningful parts of my college experience. I pledged Alpha Gamma Delta sorority and later became a Pi Kappa Alpha little sister. My fraternity brothers felt like an extension of my own, protective, welcoming, and kind. I never experienced anything close to the troubling fraternity stories that make headlines today. Murray State was safe and warm, full of people who felt like extended family. My sorority sisters were among the best friends I ever had, and that sense of belonging helped me grow up. I credit a large part of those memories to being part of Alpha Gam, and I'm still in contact with, and travel alongside, many of those same sisters nearly 40 years later.

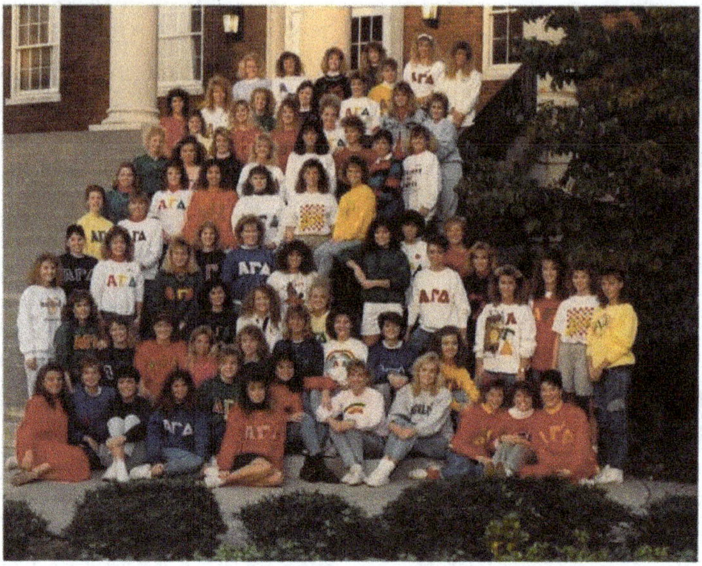

Circa 1989 – Alpha Gamma Delta Sorority, Murray State University

After that coveted internship, I returned to Murray State to finish my degree, earning a Bachelor of Science in Journalism. Academically, I was not exactly the student my parents had hoped for. My brothers had set the bar quite high. One made straight A's. Another earned both an undergraduate and a master's degree. My youngest completed two undergraduate degrees. And then there was me, who did just enough to graduate. I knew I could have done more, but I was in too much of a hurry. Too eager to start my life. Too eager to become financially independent. Too eager to move to Florida and find out what I could do on my own.

I loved journalism. I did the work. I met the deadlines. But I had held myself back, and I knew it. That quiet, nagging sense of *I could have done better* stayed with me for years and eventually became the personal push that sent me back to school for two master's degrees. This time, it wasn't about anyone else's expectations. It was about mine. I earned straight A's in every single course because I demanded it of myself.

And then there was my Doc, Dr. Robert McGaughey, my journalism professor at Murray State, my mentor, my guide, and my friend for decades. We stayed close until he passed in 2019. He even came to hear me speak at a Kentucky Breast Cancer luncheon about breast cancer survivorship and my journey as a patented inventor of a medical device for breast cancer patients. A professor and academic advisor, cheering me on more than thirty years later, I still can't quite get over that. He never stopped teaching, either. His core belief was consistent and clear: journalism isn't just about stories. It's about educating people, giving readers tools, and giving them an understanding.

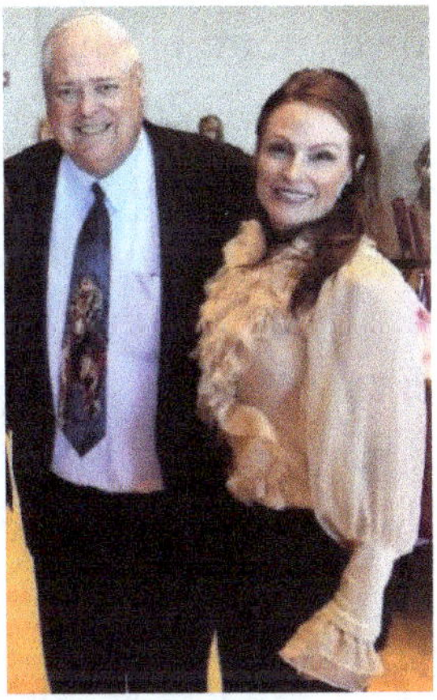

Me and Dr. Robert McGaughey, Murray State University Journalism Professor, Kentucky Breast Cancer Luncheon, 2019

My father, too, had a few core beliefs that he repeated so often they became part of me. One of them was simple, clear, and impossible to forget: buy land. Other fathers might say, *"Save your money,"* or *"Be kind to people."* My father said, *"Land is gold, Lisa. They're not making any more of it."* He said it while wiping his hands on his overalls, squinting at the sky, or staring at a crop like it was a symphony only he could hear. And he was right.

That advice stayed with me. I was 35 when I bought my first farm. One morning, while staying with my father, I was woken up by that familiar urgency in his voice. "*Lisa*," he said, *"the family down the road is auctioning off their farm. Do you want to bid on it?"*

Minutes later, we were barreling down the road in his truck. My heart was pounding, my hands sweaty. The auction was chaos: the crowd shouting, the auctioneer talking a mile a minute, bids flying from every direction. My father stood beside me, steady and silent, a rock in the storm. Then suddenly he said, *"Lisa, this land is going well under market value. Raise your hand!"* So, I did, and the next thing I knew, I was sitting at a card table inside a small travel trailer, signing papers. Just like that, it was mine. I was a farm owner, following the very rule he had drilled into my brothers and me since childhood.

Since then, I have purchased a second farm. My father is still deeply involved, guiding me through contracts, advising me on decisions, and helping me navigate a world he mastered decades ago. He is brilliant with land in a way most people can only admire from afar. Even now, with his own farms to manage, he takes the time to help me. That generosity, that knowledge, is something I carry with me every day.

My family was never content with staying in one place. My parents made sure we saw more than rows of soybeans and cornfields. Every winter, we piled into the car and drove west to Colorado. Those trips are some of my most treasured memories: mountains so impossibly tall they didn't look real, snow so deep it swallowed our boots, and my father skiing like a robot. Straight-backed, stiff, determined. We laughed at him endlessly. My mother scolded us constantly. And yet, those moments feel like pure magic when I think back on them.

On the slopes, my brothers and I developed our own language. *"Left! Right! Left!"* we would shout at every curve. My father, focused and oblivious, often missed the turn entirely. He had the worst hearing and flatly refused to purchase a hearing aid, so he would take the wrong path entirely, then curse each of us while side-stepping all the way back up the mountain to find us. We fell, we slid, we hit trees, and we made more than a few emergency room visits. My younger brother Charles seemed to collect stitches like souvenirs on most trips. We laughed until our ribs hurt. Those were the best years. The six of us moving together like one unit, laughing through every tumble, every mishap, every joyful, chaotic moment.

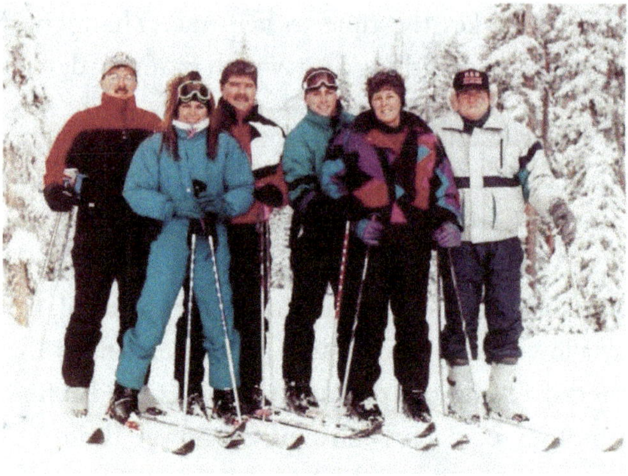

The Crites Family on the ski slopes in Colorado

My brothers and I stayed unusually close, partly because none of us rushed into marriage. Most of us married later, if at all. That meant the things we loved as children, boating, skiing, cruising, traveling, laughing, continued well into our forties. We were companions, teammates, a family that never outgrew itself.

And my mother made those years warm. She had a magical way of knowing exactly what you needed, often before you knew it yourself. She would call out of the blue and say, *"Lisa, go to page thirty of the new Victoria's Secret catalogue."* Confused, I would flip to the page, and she would say, *"I just ordered those pajamas for you. They'll be at your house in three days."* Thoughtful. Generous. Loving. Always present.

It wasn't until college that I truly realized how vast the world was. Sure, we had traveled to Tennessee to visit cousins, to Washington D.C. to learn American history, and to Colorado for ski trips. But the real awakening came during a spring break trip to the Cayman Islands to visit a childhood girlfriend. I was twenty-one, stepping off the plane, staring at beaches that looked like postcards, thinking: there is so much more out here than Missouri, Tennessee, and Kentucky. That trip planted the seed of wanderlust that has followed me ever since.

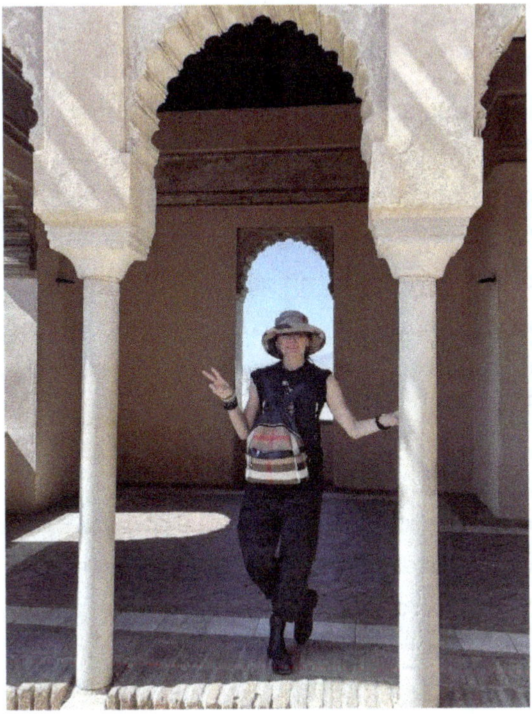

Visiting a Castle in Spain

To date, I have traveled to more than 83 countries, including seven in Asia, while working on this book.

And then there was my love life. Let's just say my early experiences with romance were lacking. In high school, even in my junior and senior years, I went to prom with friends, boys I had known since kindergarten, but I never dated seriously.

College wasn't much different. I had plenty of male friends, but my focus was on social life and figuring out who I was. Romance was never my priority.

Then, in my senior year, I met someone. He was a sophomore, two years younger, and I knew right away the timing was off. I had just turned twenty-one, and the relationship became more serious than it should have. I was deeply in love, but our lives were on different tracks. We dated for more than a year, sharing the kind of innocent, youthful joy that makes your chest feel light even as it flutters with uncertainty. After graduation, it ended. I was navigating post-college life, trying to find myself and break into journalism. During that stretch, I even worked overseas in both England and Ireland, but my heart was always set on Orlando, Florida, and health and medical journalism, the field I had always dreamed of.

We reconnected a few years later, when I was twenty-five, but nothing had changed. The timing was still wrong. I was building my life and discovering my independence, while he was buried in medical school, following in the footsteps of his father and grandfather. The problem was not a lack of love. It was there, undeniable. But life had other plans. I experienced heartbreak twice with the same person: once at twenty-two, and again at twenty-six.

After graduating from college, I moved to Florida and was hired by Walt Disney World, working as a lifeguard and picking up part-time shifts at MGM Studios. Soon after, I completed a few contracts as a fitness director for Disney Cruise Lines, which meant extensive travel up and down the eastern and western Caribbean. That experience came in handy when I began reporting for the Travel Channel.

All along, though, I was still dreaming bigger: Orlando, top 20 media market, television news. While doing segments for the Travel Channel and reporting for a local business show on Channel 6, I kept my eye on that goal. At twenty-seven, I finally got the call I had been waiting for. News director Robin Smythe hired me to cover health and medical news full-time for Channel 13. That moment was a dream realized.

My passion for medical journalism has never left me. Most television news stations chase ratings, fires, crimes, and the next political scoop, but my heart was always in health, medical, and homeopathic wellness stories. It was never just about reporting. It was about learning, understanding, and then teaching. Over the years, I have written columns for Florida Today, USA Today, The Huffington Post, Elysian Magazine, Pure Living Nashville, the Osceola News Gazette, the Orlando Sentinel, and many other platforms, covering everything from the psychology of obesity and mental health, to biohacking, neuromuscular therapy, upper cervical care, breast cancer, and both alternative and allopathic medicine. I have always included expert voices: medical doctors, surgeons, chiropractors, and psychiatrists, because clinical accuracy matters above all else. Readers have written to tell me that my columns helped them better understand eating disorders, cervical spine issues, and even the science behind donating blood. Those responses remind me that journalism, at its core, is education, and if a column can support the health of even one reader, then every hour of research is worth it.

That overwhelming curiosity eventually pulled me away from journalism and into the corporate world of medicine, and ultimately back into the classroom. After years of news deadlines, I wanted to understand the business side of healthcare. So, I took a deliberate hiatus from journalism and worked for two large multi hospital health systems as a media strategist and corporate spokesperson. In that role, it was my job to place the organization in the best light possible with the media, which in turn would gain positive newspaper, magazine, and television features. It was always a balancing act. Medicine is not perfect, humans are not perfect, and mistakes are made. So, strategy comes into play, especially when it comes to medical misadventures. I would often call my job a 'news issue management' position because I never knew what issue would pop up from day to day, needing to be managed within the Central Florida media market.

My theory was simple: keep the messaging clean, clear, concise, and tell the truth. Create strategies to communicate the issue while rectifying the problem, long before it becomes a crisis.

It's a challenging role as you must balance the media's expectations of open, full, disclosure of facts with the organization's fear of adverse publicity, while also maintaining patient confidentiality.

One time, nursery attendants gave the wrong baby to the wrong mother for breastfeeding. That was clearly not an easy story to overcome within the local media, but I had to stand tall, in front of the cameras, admit the mistake, how we would mitigate such actions from ever happening again, and move on.

Another time, a surgeon operated on the wrong limb. Again, not an easy story to overcome. But, as a media strategist, you show grace, whether you are right or wrong. In turn, you create trust and loyalty within those relationships. This work on the corporate level gave me the insight that I was craving in healthcare authenticity. I wanted to be in the middle of it, versus reporting from the outside. I have such respect for those clinicians on the hospital floor each day, taking care of patients. I believe God creates those souls to be servants' hearts, in keeping patients calm, safe, and comfortable during some of life's most vulnerable times.

My goal was never to leave news permanently. I simply wanted to understand the regulatory and transactional side of healthcare, the world behind the clinical stories I had spent years covering. That experience let me see the industry from the inside, and when I returned to print journalism, it gave me a broader, more informed perspective.

I went on to earn an MBA, then a second master's degree in digital marketing and e-commerce from the European Business School in Barcelona, Spain. Those programs educated me far more deeply than my undergraduate degree ever had. The curriculum was international, and I found myself doing case studies on companies from every corner of the world. The research sharpened my critical thinking, challenged my strategic instincts, and taught me that reinvention is not just something you do for your career. It is something you do for yourself. Most recently, Kennedy University awarded me an honorary Doctor of Philosophy in Media Communication. After more than three decades in media and journalism, that recognition felt like a quiet culmination, a moment of genuine, calming pride.

CHAPTER 2

When Life Turns on a Dime

By the time I turned 34, my career had stabilized, and my personal life seemed to finally catch up. In January 2001, I was engaged. My family was overjoyed, joking that someone had finally agreed to take me off their hands. For the first time, I allowed myself to envision a life of balance: love, an extended family, and career coexisting in harmony. But life, as it so often does, had other plans.

Within a month of my engagement, my father was rushed into emergency surgery. He had been diagnosed with Mallory-Weiss syndrome, a rare condition affecting roughly seven in 100,000 people, involving a torn artery in his esophagus. The situation was critical. He spent six weeks in the ICU, with doctors warning that even if he survived, he might be left in a vegetative state. For six weeks, our family lived inside that hospital, clinging to faith when medical prognoses offered little hope. By the grace of God, he made a full recovery: no brain damage, no memory loss, no long-term effects. It felt miraculous, as if divine hands had intervened.

My mother had returned from a shopping trip in Memphis when she noticed brown stains on my father's shirt. When she asked, he said he had vomited blood. Within minutes, he began vomiting again, and she called 911. An ambulance rushed him to the nearest hospital, even though his condition required a trauma center that was too far away. Emergency surgery revealed the Mallory-Weiss tear. Doctors were initially baffled, asking whether my father drank, as the condition is more common in alcoholics due to a weakened esophagus. He barely drank at all. This was a freak occurrence, a rare medical anomaly. During surgery, he flatlined. The team was direct: survival would be a miracle, and if he lived, he would never be the same. My mother, my brothers, and I quietly began discussing what life might look like if he did survive.

He remained in a medically induced coma in the ICU for weeks. The medical team attempted to remove the intubation tube once, but he was combative, throwing a nurse across the bed, and they put him back under. They tried again after another ten days.

When they removed the intubation tube for the second time, I followed the advice of my fiancé, an orthopedic clinician, who flew to the Midwest to help guide clinical decisions. He told me to sit beside my father and talk to him continuously, even without a response. I spoke to him for thirty-six hours straight, asking every conceivable question: trucks he had driven, his birthdate, his children, reminding him who he was, who we were, who I was. At first, he did not recognize me, only acknowledging that he had a daughter who worked in television news. The environment was cold, clinical, and tense, but I persisted. The trauma center that could have provided more resources was an hour away, and my father was too unstable to transfer for weeks. And yet, against all odds, God's hands were unmistakable in his recovery.

Within days, he returned to baseline: fully alive, fully present, a living testament to physical and mental resilience and divine intervention. After that medical scare, my father chose to retire at 62 years of age.

A few months later, in November 2001, my fiancé and I were married. It was a beautiful wedding, adorned with Christmas decorations, red velvet, live poinsettias, laughter, and hope. Friends and family traveled in from all over, including England, Ireland, and Germany, to celebrate with us. There was a collective exhale in the room, a shared belief that happiness had finally found me.

We met because he was my orthopedic provider, from a shoulder injury I sustained while covering hurricanes for the news station. We dated a little over a year before marrying. He was considerate, thoughtful, and supportive. I soon expected to be settling into my new life, an extended honeymoon period.

But, to the contrary, there are catastrophes that don't knock. They just walk straight in and take over the room...and your life.

Two weeks after my wedding, my world shattered. I still feel the emotion of writing these words, still hesitate, as if, more than two decades later, it might somehow not be true. But it is. That is when I lost my mother. Just like that. A car accident. One moment, she was alive and busy decorating for Christmas, and the next, she was gone. Sixty years old. Full of energy. Full of plans. She had only recently become a grandmother.

I don't think anyone can fully understand how a single phone call can split a life into a before and an after. But that one did.

My husband and I had only been home from our honeymoon for one day. I remember calling her to say we had made it back safely. I told her I had caught the flu. We laughed about my timing. That was it. That was our last conversation. The next morning, my phone rang. It was my brother Shawn. I knew something was wrong before he even spoke. He told me she had been in an accident. He told me she was gone. I don't remember screaming. I don't even remember breathing. I only remember the room tilting.

Within minutes, my husband walked through the door, still in his surgical cap and booties. He had received an emergency call from my family and rushed straight to me. I had been a bride home from her honeymoon one moment and a grieving, motherless daughter the next. I didn't even have time to catch up with my own joy before grief swallowed me whole.

It was December 19th. Eight days after her birthday. One of those bitter cold Midwest days where the sky hangs low and grey, as if it already knows what's coming. She had left the house to meet friends. Half a mile from our family farm. Half a mile. That was all.

My father, well known in the area for his philanthropic efforts and decades on the school board, accidentally drove upon the scene. He was stopped by a state patrolman who said, *"Mr. Crites, we have some bad news. Your wife had an accident and died on the scene. You will need to identify her body."*

After 42 years of marriage, I don't know how a person endures a sentence like that.

The last time I saw my mother was on my wedding day. That is the image I carry. Even now, I keep wedding photos around the house. My second husband, David, understands why. That day was the last time our family was whole. I remember trying to call her the morning of the accident, and she didn't answer. I assumed she was outside walking her dogs. Within an hour, she was gone. She had left our farmhouse for Christmas brunch with her girlfriends, crossed Highway 60, a main thoroughfare in the Midwest, and was struck by a college student driving home for Christmas break. She was not wearing her seatbelt, and the impact ejected her from the SUV. She landed on the side of the road with a broken collarbone.

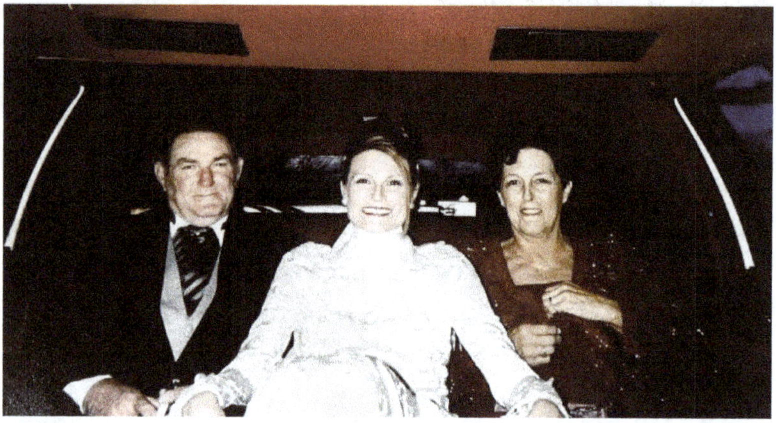

My Dad, me, and My Mother
(the last time I saw my mother, the evening of my wedding)

The news of it feels unreal even now, like I am talking about someone else's mother.

A school bus full of high school students witnessed the scene. One of them had just learned CPR and tried to help her, not realizing she had already passed. That detail still breaks me in a way I cannot fully explain. Someone trying so hard. And it was already too late.

My father, strong as stone and stubborn as the earth itself, the man I have always described as John Wayne with a little Archie Bunker, had to step forward and say, *"Yes, that's my wife."* I caught the next flight from Florida, and when I saw him the following day, I asked what my mother looked like lying on the ground. I don't know why I asked. Part of me needed the truth. Another part needed comfort. And in some ways, I was doing what journalists do: asking the hard question because not knowing felt worse. He said she was lying with one arm over her head, like she was sleeping. No visible injuries, except for blood from one ear. He said it looked like she never knew what hit her. Instant. Fast. Merciful in its own terrible way.

That image still follows me. It haunts me. But strangely, it also comforts me.

A few days later, we retrieved her personal belongings from the impounded SUV. Inside, we found dozens of individually initialed Christmas bracelets she had bought for her friends. I delivered them over the following days. It was one of the hardest things I have ever done, and also one of the most sacred.

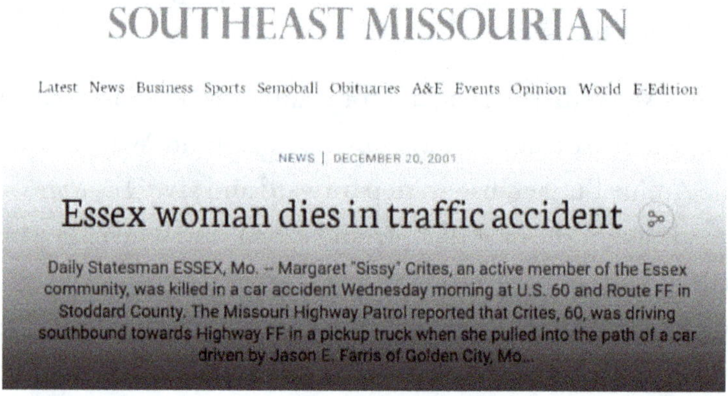
SOUTHEAST MISSOURIAN

Latest News Business Sports Semoball Obituaries A&E Events Opinion World E-Edition

NEWS | DECEMBER 20, 2001

Essex woman dies in traffic accident

Daily Statesman ESSEX, Mo. -- Margaret "Sissy" Crites, an active member of the Essex community, was killed in a car accident Wednesday morning at U.S. 60 and Route FF in Stoddard County. The Missouri Highway Patrol reported that Crites, 60, was driving southbound towards Highway FF in a pickup truck when she pulled into the path of a car driven by Jason E. Farris of Golden City, Mo...

Newspaper Clipping Of My Mother's Fatal Accident

My mother's death changed me. It changed the dynamics of our entire family. My brothers were in their own pain. My father was in his. And I was in mine. Over the years, we have grown apart, which grieves me still. Death has a way of doing that: changing the people you love most, and changing how you love them. When everyone is searching for their new normal, relationships shift, and sometimes they dissolve.

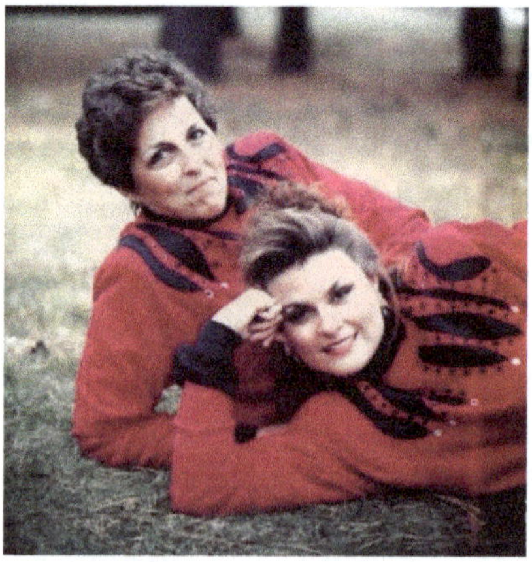

Me and My Mother

Even now, I don't fully understand why God took my mother at 60. I am 59. That confusion still sits quietly inside me. But somewhere in the middle of all that darkness, I felt something else too. At the funeral home, in the heaviness and the shock, I felt a quiet, steady presence guiding me. Not loud. Not dramatic. Just steady. Clear.

The months that followed were brutal. I was in a new marriage, a new house, a new life, and yet I felt like I was drowning. I felt helpless and overwhelmed. Grief and severe depression wrapped around me like a fog I could not find my way out of.

I took family medical leave from work and retreated to the Midwest, staying with my father for three long months. I exercised. I read. I cried. I slept. I cleaned out my mother's belongings. My childhood friends were my constant companions through that cold winter, and they understood what I had lost in a way few people could. They had always joked that the umbilical cord between my mother and me was never really cut. They knew she had always been my best friend.

I was so focused on rebuilding myself that I did everything I could to stay healthy, including not touching alcohol for an entire year. Friends suggested I needed to relax and take the edge off, but I knew better. I needed to guard my mind, body, and spirit carefully. Unhealthy habits were luxuries I could not afford when my psychological survival felt so fragile.

Two books became my lifeline. The first was *Motherless Daughters: The Legacy of Loss* by Hope Edelman, gifted to me at my mother's funeral by my friend April Wilson. April was a licensed social worker who had lost her own mother young. She knew what my future was going to look like before I did. Nearly twenty-five years later, I still have that book, and the handwritten message April left inside it.

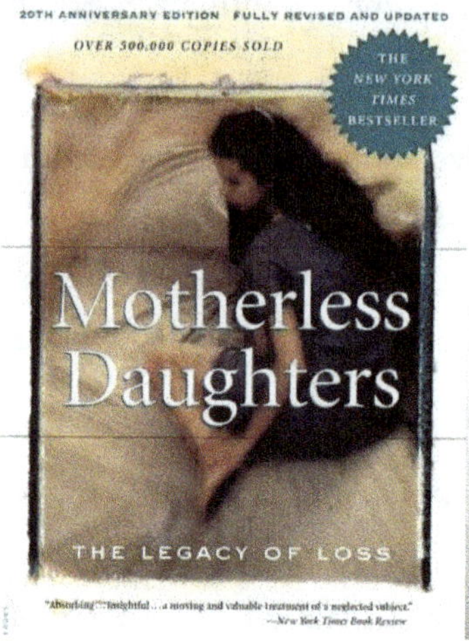

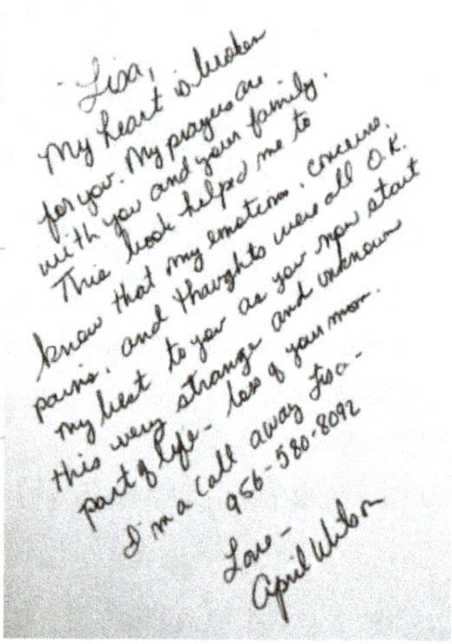

Edelman wrote *Motherless Daughters* after spending decades reflecting on the profound impact of losing her mother during her teenage years. Her words illuminated the deep scars that losing a mother imprints on a daughter. They validated my experience, gave voice to my grief, and offered some small comfort. Yet even with that guidance, I still wrestled with insecurity, self-doubt, and the nagging fear that I might never have the strength to truly navigate the emotions surrounding my mother's loss.

The second lifeline was *Talking to Heaven* by James Van Praagh, a writer I had long admired. Van Praagh is a self-described medium who affirms his belief in a peaceful afterlife and offers perspectives on healthy grieving. I believe I read that book at least five times.

My husband at the time, the first David, was a kind and caring man, but he didn't understand the depth of my sadness. He kept telling me I should be further along in the grieving process than I was. I remember thinking: maybe something is wrong with me. Maybe I'm not strong enough to survive losing my mother. It took me a while to realize it wasn't psychological weakness. It was trauma.

The mental anguish was intense. Some weeks, the pain was so unbearable that I would sleep for days at a stretch. Eight months after my mother's accident, I finally sought grief therapy. I will never forget what my counselor told me, a truth I have since shared with countless others navigating immediate loss. She explained that a person cannot begin the grieving and mourning process until they are no longer in a state of trauma. She described how the brain reacts to sudden death: the trauma itself blocks the proper grieving process, and it could take a year or more before the mind can truly begin to process the loss. That was a profound revelation. It helped. But I knew I still had a long way to go.

My marriage, unfortunately, could not withstand the storm. In 2006, after five years together, we divorced. Looking back, it made sense. Within two weeks of saying *"I do,"* we had been confronted with unimaginable tragedy, and we simply didn't have enough foundation to survive the peaks and valleys that followed. Within that same period, his mother passed away, and then my mother's brother, Uncle Joe, my cousin Mandy's father, died a few months after that. Three major losses in a year and a half. Another wave of grief. Another hit to an already fragile emotional state.

He meant well, he truly did. He wanted me to feel better. But he didn't know how to sit with my sorrow. He wanted to appear strong and untouched by the chaos, and in trying to be that, he retreated. I don't believe he meant any harm, but life, grief, and circumstances outweighed the marriage in ways love alone couldn't fix. I know he was struggling too, because he had loved my mother. But our marriage couldn't hold the weight of my grief, and that became the fracture line. We separated after four years, and a year later, the divorce was finalized.

When I moved out, I finally began to breathe again. I bought a downtown condo in Orlando, and for the first time since my mother's accident, I felt clarity returning. A sense of myself returning. The weight of that marriage lifted, along with the suffocating grief I had been carrying like a stone in my chest. My aunt once asked me gently, *"Do you think your marriage might have worked if you had been married longer, and had children, before your mother died?"* I thought about it honestly, and the answer was no. Our foundation had been too fragile. The divorce was painful, but it became a necessary step toward my own healing.

I remember thinking during that time: I am 39, approaching 40, and going through a divorce. I felt like a colossal failure. Divorce was not something I had witnessed in my family. My grandparents had stayed together until their deaths. My parents had been married for 42 years before my mother died. I felt as though I had let my family down, as though I had failed to live up to an unspoken legacy of stability and endurance.

Before my mother's passing, I was strong and independent, but also high-strung and quick to let life's hardships cut deep. Losing her taught me something I hadn't expected: how to blend strength with softness. Her sweet and caring nature had always been a steady light in our family. I had always leaned toward my father's practicality and no-nonsense logic. But grief has a way of rearranging you. Losing her taught me to combine resilience with empathy, power with compassion.

After my divorce, I swore I would never marry again. Marriage had cast a long shadow, and I was determined to focus on myself: my growth, my independence, my life. And yet life has a way of surprising you when you least expect it.

My second husband entered my life quietly, not as a romantic interest, at least not at first. I knew him as a friend. He was the corporate attorney for the hospital system where I worked as a media strategist. I saw him in meetings, watched him navigate litigation, and quietly admired his intelligence, his insight, his presence. I got to know him better through his executive assistant, and one of my closest friends, Susie, and realized quickly that he was the kind of person you could trust; someone who observes carefully, listens intently, and remembers. For seven years, we were simply friends.

Our foundation was built on respect, but what made me fall in love with him was something deeper. He talked to me about my mother. He could acknowledge my grief without flinching, without turning away. He was patient, compassionate, and present. He didn't try to fix anything. He didn't shy away from my pain. He honored it. And in that honoring, I found myself opening in ways I never had before.

Our friendship gradually deepened into love, and eventually into marriage. He had been through his own losses and rebuilding, so he understood what that looked like. More than that, he embraced my family, my history, and the memory of my mother. He never knew her personally, yet he spoke of her with warmth, as if he had. That respect made all the difference. It reassured me that grief could live alongside love, that one doesn't cancel out the other.

In him, I found a partner who could hold space for my past while walking with me into the future. A love built on friendship, shared experience, and a genuine understanding of the heart. In 2013, after 15 years of friendship and eight years together, we married. His name is also David, though I call him Phil, based on his resemblance to Phil Donahue, which also helpfully resolves the confusion of having married two men with the same name.

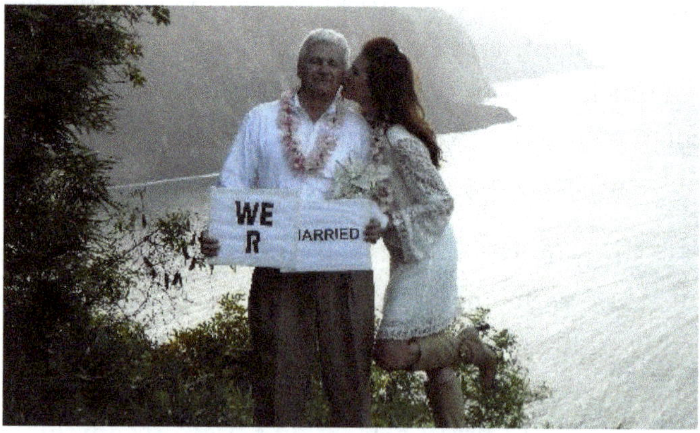

Me and Phil married in Hawaii

CHAPTER 3

The Diagnosis and the Decision

Years passed as I struggled to find my way through the grief of losing my mother and the wreckage of a divorce. I was still trying to put myself back together when, in 2009, life delivered another shattering blow.

It was the second most traumatic day of my life.

Nearly eight years after my mother's death, I found myself standing in that exact same headspace: traumatized, overwhelmed, and plagued by a feeling of helplessness and loss of control. This time, it wasn't a death that had brought me to my knees. It was a diagnosis that was about to change the trajectory of my health, life, and career.

I had breast cancer.

I went completely numb. Blank. Confused. I was the medical reporter who interviewed breast cancer patients, not the one sitting in their chair. I didn't know what to do, where to turn, or how to begin processing what was happening. It felt like every aspect of my spirit was being tested again.

It started with a lump in my right breast. For years, like most women, I had been told to do self-breast exams, but no one ever really explained what I was supposed to be feeling for, so I never made it a consistent habit. It always felt vague, almost abstract, until one day it wasn't.

I was interviewing a breast surgeon when he said something that stayed with me. He explained that when you check regularly, you don't need to be an expert. You simply learn what feels normal for your body, and you notice when something changes. That was the moment it clicked.

I started doing self-exams, not obsessively, just consistently. Over the next four or five months, everything felt the same. Then, by the sixth month, it didn't. There was a lump in my right breast, unmistakable and new. I knew immediately it hadn't been there before, and in that moment, my life quietly shifted in a way I could not yet understand.

As any proactive woman would do, I made an appointment with my OB/GYN, who immediately referred me for a mammogram. I went through the usual motions, not thinking too much of it. You tell yourself it's probably nothing: a cyst, hormone fluctuations, a fluke. You cling to optimism because everyone says that staying positive is the key. But when the radiologist began studying the images, the temperature in the room seemed to drop. I could sense his concern.

It wasn't the lump itself that worried him. It was a cluster of calcifications tucked behind it. He compared the new scans to my mammograms from the previous three years and identified a troubling trend: those calcifications hadn't just grown, they had multiplied. He looked at me and said he wanted to schedule a biopsy for the following week. I tried to stay calm. I really did. But deep down, a part of me already knew.

Ever since I was a little girl, I have experienced a series of recurring dreams: visions that I would eventually be diagnosed with breast cancer. At the time, I didn't understand them. I assumed I simply had a creative imagination fueled by fear. But I had also dreamed, repeatedly, that my mother would die tragically. That nightmare had already become reality, and I had begun taking my premonitions far more seriously. It was why I was so diligent about scheduling those annual mammograms. In some part of myself, I had been waiting for the other shoe to drop.

The day after the biopsy, my phone rang. It was the surgeon. His tone was kind, but there was an urgency beneath it that made my stomach turn slowly. He asked if we could move my follow-up appointment from the following week to the very next day. I didn't need to be a doctor to understand what that meant.

At the time, I was in the middle of one of my journalism hiatuses, working as Director of Media Strategy for a large multi-hospital system in Central Florida. It happened to be the very same hospital where my biopsy had been performed. Because I had access to medical records, I decided I wasn't going to sit and wait for a formal appointment to hear what I already suspected.

I walked straight to the medical records department and picked up my report. I remember holding that piece of paper, my hands trembling slightly, scanning the medical language until my eyes locked onto the words printed in bold: Patient has Ductal Carcinoma in Situ (DCIS) in the right breast.

As a medical reporter, I had interviewed countless breast cancer patients. I knew exactly what those words meant.

For a moment, the world just stopped. My mind froze. My heart hammered against my ribs. I could barely catch my breath. In a strange cocktail of denial and disbelief, I walked straight to the Emergency Department to find my friend Stephen Beyer, who managed the department. I shoved the report into his hands and asked him to read it. I think I was hoping that my eyes, and my years of medical journalism, had somehow failed me, that I had misread some technicality.

He looked at the paper, then looked back at me, and said softly, *"Lisa, you're reading it correctly. You have breast cancer."*

I didn't stop there. I found another friend, a physician, who confirmed the same. And then I kept going. I wandered the hospital hallways in a total daze, medical report in hand, like a ghost haunting my own workplace. Every few minutes, I would stop a nurse, a doctor, anyone I knew who could read medical terminology, asking them to just double-check. Each one looked at me with the same quiet, sympathetic expression and nodded. Yes. Breast cancer.

The bottom line was that we were all reading English, and we all knew what the report said. Stephen and I still laugh about that day: the image of me desperately roaming those halls, waiting for someone, anyone, to tell me I didn't have cancer. Unfortunately, those words were not spoken that afternoon.

When you're a child, and fear creeps in, you run to your mother without thinking. She is your safe place, your calm in the chaos. But when fear found me this time, there was nowhere to run. My mother, the woman who had always steadied me in every storm, was no longer there. That absence pressed down on me just as hard as the diagnosis itself.

All I could think was: I just want to take a nap.

Napping is my default. It is my Blue Screen of Death restart. Everyone who knows me, my family, my friends, my colleagues, knows that when my world feels like it is crashing, I go to sleep. It is my way of pressing pause when life feels too big to manage.

I walked back to my office, still in a daze, those words swirling in my head like a storm. I sat at my desk, opened my email, and typed a message to my inner circle:

"I have breast cancer. I will be out of contact for a few days. DO NOT worry, but I will be in touch. I am fine, but I do not want to talk about this right now. I am turning my cell phone off, and I need to go home and take a nap!!!"

I hit send, shut off my phone, and walked out. My friends and family still mock me over that email. They were worried and frustrated that I had dropped a bomb that bluntly and then simply vanished. But in that moment, it was the only way I knew how to cope.

Within a week, my life became a blur of sterile offices and hospital corridors. I was hunting for second opinions, and every doctor had a different piece of advice. The options were clear, but they were all terrifying.

Option 1: A lumpectomy to clear the margins, followed by six weeks of chemotherapy and radiation, then five years of Tamoxifen.

Option 2: A unilateral mastectomy, the removal of the compromised breast, with the possibility of reconstruction.

Option 3: A bilateral mastectomy, the total removal of both breasts, with the possibility of reconstruction.

I tried to visualize myself living through each choice. All were difficult. I couldn't fathom radiating my chest or having chemotherapy running through my veins. I had spent decades caring for my body: exercising, eating well, monitoring what I put into it. The idea of medicinal poison coursing through me felt unacceptable, both emotionally and psychologically. Yet I knew it might be a clinical requirement, a step I might not have a choice in.

I didn't want this disease to define my life a second longer than it had to. If I chose the lumpectomy, I knew I would spend every subsequent year in a low hum of panic, waiting for a recurrence. Every morning I swallowed a Tamoxifen pill; I would be reminded that I was a cancer patient. That wasn't the life I wanted.

I had known too many women with breast cancer. I had served on the board of directors of a national breast cancer support group and witnessed firsthand what happened when the disease returned. Recurrence never came quietly. It came back unyielding, more aggressive, almost as if it had something to prove. I had seen the toll it took on their bodies, their families, and their hope. I didn't want to give my cancer that kind of second chance.

I recognized quickly which path felt right for me. A bilateral mastectomy would allow me to take control, protect my body from the poisons of treatment, and preserve the part of myself that mattered most. It would also mean that by removing both breasts, my chances of the cancer returning decreased exponentially. And if it came down to losing my hair or my breasts, the choice was clear: my connection to my hair ran deeper than any emotional attachment to my breasts.

For me, it wasn't just a medical decision. It was a psychological one. Every breast cancer patient must choose what is emotionally acceptable for her. What feels right for one woman might feel like a tragedy to another. For me, a bilateral mastectomy was the only path that offered a genuine sense of reclaiming control in a situation that had made me feel powerless.

I remember a lengthy conversation with my Aunt Faye, my namesake, Lisa Faye. At 75, she had these glamorous, voluptuous, Marilyn Monroe-style breasts, and she told me she could never imagine living without them. *"They are a part of who I am,"* she said.

Listening to her, I recognized a real generational divide in how we viewed our bodies. Women of her era were often defined by their femininity in an extremely specific, physical way. But for me, it was different. I had grown up with three brothers on a farm, racing motorcycles through the mud, and I had never been drawn to that version of femininity. Sports bras were my choice. I was a tomboy, rarely wearing dresses, much to the dismay of my mother and my two elegantly dressed grandmothers.

I told her, *"Aunt Faye, I'm not really that in touch with my femininity. I just need to get rid of this diseased breast. And I'm far more emotionally connected to my hair than to my breasts, so if something has to go, it's going to be the breasts every time."*

She laughed and shook her head. She didn't quite understand it, but she respected it. She accepted that for me, this was not a loss. It was freedom. It was my way of ending the hold this disease had on me and stepping into the next chapter on my own terms.

Even knowing I was making the right decision, the emotional and psychological weight of it was grueling, and the complications that followed were relentless: infections, unexpected surgeries, setbacks that arrived before the last ones had healed. Yet I endured each one, step by step, because I had already survived a pain far deeper. Losing my mother had reshaped the very core of who I was, and learning to survive that had quietly prepared me to survive this. Knowledge, preparation, and an inner fortitude I hadn't known I possessed carried me through what turned out to be a long and clinically complex reconstruction journey.

The complications hit hard and fast. Just ten days after surgery, a fever of 104 degrees in the middle of the night told me something was very wrong. The tissue expander and wound on the left side had become severely infected. Cellulitis had set in, spreading through the deeper layers of my skin. I still had post-surgical drains in place, and my body was literally pushing the infection out through those tubes. When the emergency room doctor examined my chest, he told me plainly that without those drains, I would likely have gone into septic shock. Bloodwork confirmed how serious it was: my white blood cell count had climbed to 18,000. And it wasn't only cellulitis. Tests also revealed Methicillin-resistant Staphylococcus, MRSA.

I spent twelve days in the hospital while clinicians cycled through antibiotics trying to resolve the infection, with no success. I underwent removal of the left tissue expander, repeated surgeries, and months of hyperbaric oxygen treatments. Fourteen months. Seven surgeries. Two infections. Every day felt like a test. Every shower, a challenge. And all the while, I tried to keep my media work afloat on part-time hours and short-term disability, clinging to some sense of purpose and normalcy.

By 41, I had now lived through two events that were, each in their own way, unimaginable. The first was losing my mother and everything that unraveled in the years that followed. The second was this: a cancer diagnosis, a radical surgery, and a recovery that tested me in ways I had never anticipated. Both had changed me permanently. And somehow, improbably, I was still standing.

The diagnosis was, in many ways, statistically improbable. Only one percent of women in the United States receive a breast cancer diagnosis in their early forties. I was healthy. I did not smoke, rarely drank, exercised daily, and took exceptional care of myself. There was no history of breast cancer in my family. And yet those words, *"you have breast cancer,"* remain unimaginable for a thousand distinct reasons.

But here is the kicker. When the pathology report came back after my mastectomy, it revealed that I had cancer in both breasts, not just the right one. The left breast showed lobular carcinoma in situ (LCIS), indicating abnormal cells on a path toward a more aggressive, invasive cancer.

I remember speaking with my surgeon after the surgery, genuinely shaken that cancer had been present in both. He looked at me and said, *"Lisa, the cancer is gone."*

I told him that wasn't the point. Knowledge is power, and I had lacked that knowledge. I had made the right call without even knowing the full picture.

I kept thinking: what if I had only done the lumpectomy? What if I had only had the right breast removed? I would have been living my life with aggressive cancer growing in the other one, completely unaware. And I kept returning to the theory that had guided me from the beginning: if my body had produced a diseased breast once, it could do so again. That reasoning, as it turned out, had been exactly right. Unbeknownst to me, my body had already produced two. Had I chosen differently, I would have been back in surgery months or years later, and there is no telling what stage that cancer would have reached by then.

I chose the right path. I genuinely believe God was watching over me, guiding both my decisions and my surgeon's hands, with my guardian angels close by and my mother leading that pack from somewhere just out of reach.

After enduring my mother's death, a cancer diagnosis, severe complications, multiple surgeries, and the kind of mental, physical, and psychological trauma that made me question my own resilience, I finally began to emerge from the mental darkness. But, to put it simply: a sudden, tragic loss like my mother's is never truly overcome. You learn to manage it. You learn to navigate the waves with more steadiness, more control.

Seven years after her death, sitting on a beach reading a book about grief, I finally found the words for what I had been living. The author described how sometimes you walk along the shore with waves rolling gently over your feet, slow and steady. And then, without warning, a wave crashes in fast and hard, knocking you off balance entirely.

It was the perfect metaphor. Grief comes in waves, and we spend a lifetime learning how to stand through them.

Continued counseling helped me work through the trauma of both losses: my mother's death and the physical and psychological toll of breast cancer. My counselor helped me reach a place where the grief no longer controlled me completely, where it came and went in smaller, more manageable waves.

When I reached that place, I felt stronger than I had in years. I vowed never to sink that deep again. And looking back now, I can see how much better I am because of everything I endured. I became more empathetic, more resilient, and more capable of sitting with pain, my own and other people's. That resilience is also, I believe, a large part of why I survived the complications from breast cancer as well as I did.

When I faced cancer, friends often remarked on how composed I seemed, how well I appeared to be handling it. But if I am honest, it was not the worst thing I had been through. Losing my mother was. That heartbreak came first, and it reshaped me in ways that gave me the perspective, the strength, and the steadiness to face whatever came next.

My mother's death broke me. But it also built me. And in the end, I think that is exactly what she would have wanted.

CHAPTER 4

The Truth We Tell to Survive

June 2009 is a month I vividly remember. I wasn't just having a bilateral mastectomy; I was also beginning the first stage of breast reconstruction. I remember lying in the pre-surgery room, the hum of machines filling the sterile space, the smell of antiseptic sharp in the air. A quiet tension seeped into my bones, the kind that always lingers before something life-changing. My dad was on one side of me, steady and strong, and my significant other, David (Phil), was on the other, holding my hand. Their presence should have been enough. But it wasn't.

All I could think about was my mom.

I began to cry, not because I was afraid of the surgery, but because of the deep ache of her absence. I knew it probably seemed insensitive to the two people beside me, trying so hard to offer comfort, yet I could not stop thinking about how much I needed her at that moment.

I had spent my teenage years and college days by her side, watching her endure multiple breast biopsies for calcifications and masses. Back then, mammograms used analog technology, not digital, so any visual concern required a biopsy. She had gone through at least a dozen over the years. I had sat beside her in surgical waiting rooms countless times, her hand in mine, listening as she told doctors firmly, *"If you see cancer, take them off."* Fortunately, she never had cancer. But like mother, like daughter, I had said those exact same words to my own doctor years later. Now, when I needed her most, she could not be there. That absence hit me harder than anything else that day.

I soon realized I had my 57-year-old boyfriend on one side of the bed and my 70-year-old father on the other, both in tears. A nurse walked in, took one look at them, smiled, and said, *"You guys need happy meds."*

That evening, after eight hours of surgery, I woke up in severe pain. My first words were, *"If I had known it would hurt this much, I would have chosen a lumpectomy."* The same nurse who had given me the happy meds that morning overheard me and said quietly, *"Lisa, you made the right decision."*

There isn't much time to process the reality of losing your breasts when unbearable pain becomes your only focus. The pain on the right side of my chest was so intense I could barely breathe, constant and relentless, as if an arrow had been driven straight into my breast where the cancer had been. I kept complaining about it, and my primary surgeon, Dr. John O'Linde, said, *"Lisa, the breast that had the cancer is usually the one that causes the most pain after surgery."* He was absolutely right.

The next memory is hazy, fogged by anesthesia and morphine, but vivid in emotional detail. I woke the following morning to find the fog had lifted just enough for the pain to hit again. My chest felt heavy, sore, almost foreign. I opened my eyes to see my cousin Mandy standing in the doorway. She had flown in from Kansas City early that morning.

Mandy, nearly six feet tall, blonde, always impeccably dressed, hair perfectly styled, makeup flawless. And there I was, pale and groggy, lying flat in a hospital bed. Through the haze of morphine, my first coherent thought was: Mandy looks so pretty. Oh my gosh. I have no breasts.

And then I cried.

I had never been emotionally attached to my breasts, but being able to look down and see the physical reality, the dried, bloody bandages, the stitches where my breasts once were, was shocking. The tissue expanders sutured into my chest felt odd, lumpy, almost alien. They were temporary, inflatable devices placed under the skin and muscle to stretch the tissue, creating a pocket for a permanent implant. Not soft or natural, not even like breast implants. Simply placeholders, for something that had been, and something that would eventually take months to rebuild.

That was the first moment I truly felt the weight of what had happened, and the weight of my choices. My body was forever changed.

A little while later, my reconstructive surgeon came in to examine the surgical sites. Mandy sat across the room, trying to appear calm. When the doctor removed the bandages, I watched the color drain from her face. She forced a smile, mouthing, *"Lisa, it doesn't look that bad. It doesn't look that bad."*

I wanted to believe her. But I knew she wasn't being truthful.

It took me back fifteen years, to when Mandy had skin cancer on her nose. I had gone with her after they removed the damaged tissue to begin reconstruction, a cartilage graft from her ear, sutured to rebuild the nostril. I had stood there looking at her face and said the exact same words: *"Mandy, it doesn't look that bad."* I had not told her the truth then, just as she was not telling me the truth now.

Reality hit when I finally looked in the mirror. Bewildered, pale, still disoriented from the anesthesia, I cried. And this time, Mandy cried with me.

We both knew the truth. The visual outcome of my mastectomy was deeply confronting. I thought I had prepared myself emotionally and psychologically for surgery, but the physical reality was something I had not fully faced until that moment. Any amputation of a body part is shocking. This was no different.

Mandy had always been my comfort. One year younger, yet somehow always more mature and steady, she had earned the nickname *"Mother Mandy"* among our friends. That day, she was every bit the nurturing cousin, the motherly figure, the friend I needed. I had insisted she be there from the moment I was diagnosed. Now I understand why. She filled the hole left by my mother's absence, a steady, comforting presence when I needed one most.

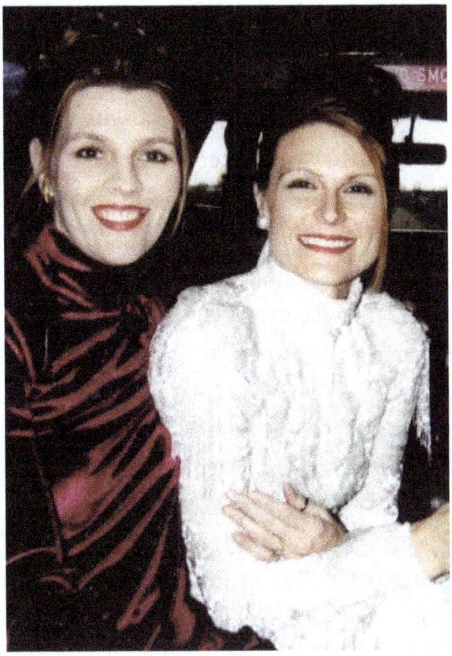

Cousin Mandy & Me

More than a year later, when I was healed and able to laugh about it, Mandy and I finally admitted the truth to each other. Neither of those visuals had *"looked okay."* Not the first time she saw me post-surgery, nor the times I had tried to reassure her about her nose. But sometimes love sounds like reassurance, even when the truth is too hard to face.

We had both been through surgeries that left scars, visible and invisible. And in hindsight, we realized that healing was not just physical. It was emotional, raw, and, if we allowed ourselves to see it, a little funny.

Under ordinary circumstances, I would have expected the initial healing process after my mastectomy to be manageable, perhaps occasionally difficult, but nothing catastrophic. My recovery, however, was far from ordinary. Clinical complications turned what should have been weeks of healing into months of uncertainty and agony. I didn't know from one day to the next whether I would ever have two breasts again.

I remember the day my surgeon said it, clear as if it were etched into my brain:

"Lisa, if you have one more infection, we will not be able to complete reconstruction. You will only have one breast for the rest of your life."

I remember thinking: that was never in the cards. That was never the plan. That was never an option. I had chosen a bilateral mastectomy with reconstruction, imagining the process unfolding the way friends had described it: surgery, then reconstruction, completion within six to eight months. Instead, reality hit like a freight train.

Despite multiple antibiotics and the best efforts of my surgical team, the MRSA would not relent. The infection had driven so deep into my chest and stomach wall that I could barely sit up or lie down on my own. My left breast, the side that had not even appeared to have cancer prior to surgery, became a battlefield. My surgeons had no choice but to remove the infected tissue expander.

The infectious disease doctor explained it in a voice that was clinical but steady:

"When you place a foreign object into your body and it becomes infected, it is compromised. We don't want to negatively affect your reconstruction or overall healing. We must remove the expander. By removing it, we can flush the tissue to support the removal of the infection. We believe this is hospital-acquired MRSA, and we are concerned it could colonize into the tissues of your chest or other regions of your body."

I sobbed. I had been hospitalized for twelve days, running high fevers, cycling between delirium and pain medication. I was desperately trying to reclaim some of the mental strength I had lost the moment I was readmitted through the emergency department. And now this setback would mean additional months of clinical processes and potentially more complications. My body felt like a betrayal.

I was lucid enough to understand that this infection had potentially altered my physical appearance for life. As I have said before, I had never been emotionally attached to my breasts, yet I had expected to regain the appearance of both after surgery. Now uncertainty hung over me like a shadow. Would the scar tissue or surgical complications prevent me from ever completing reconstruction?

When the doctor left, a nurse returned, approaching cautiously. She had that particular mix of empathy and professional hesitation that only experienced nurses develop when someone is at the brink of emotional collapse.

"Are you familiar with Xanax?" she asked gently. *"Would you like one?"*

I couldn't respond. I simply nodded. She handed it over immediately, and I swallowed it like a lifeline.

I knew enough about these types of infections to know this was the beginning of a long and complicated process. I was right.

The following morning was a Sunday, and the hospital felt like a ghost town. Empty hallways, a quiet eeriness, everything muted except for the distant sound of monitors. They rolled me back into surgery to remove the infected tissue expander. After two hours, I slept the rest of the day.

My body was inflamed and traumatized, but surprisingly, my chest no longer ached the way it had. The infection had been flushed out, the deep layers of cellulitis finally addressed. I was left with what I called an elongated rib, and a small tube tied in a knot to drain any remaining infection.

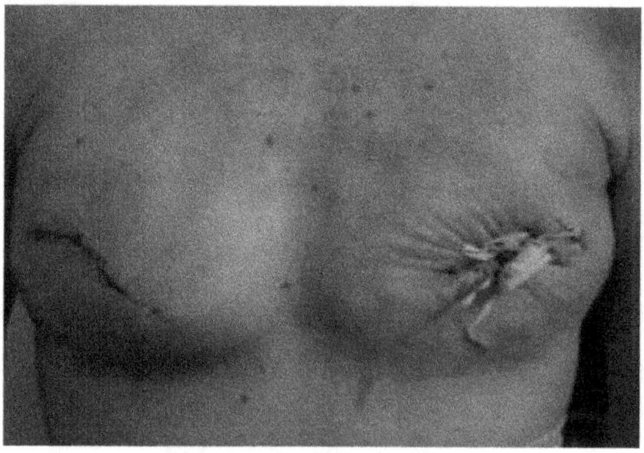

The future was uncertain, entirely dependent on how my body would heal. In the meantime, I was left both mentally and physically exhausted, without a breast on the left side of my body, only a painful, knotted drain, extensive scarring, and a single tissue expander on the right.

I often say I lost twelve days of my life in that hospital. And in truth, I did. My memory of that time is a blur, a fog of pain, fear, and relief. I remember a large, private hospital room at the end of a long hall. I remember it belonged to the same healthcare system where I worked as corporate media strategist and spokesperson, a surreal twist: a hospital-acquired infection happening to the very person who was their public face.

I remember David sitting next to the window, working quietly on his laptop. I remember my boss, Johnette, visiting and bringing me a stone cross. I remember large arrangements of flowers scattered around the room. And I remember the infectious disease doctor, firm but precise, directing the expander removal.

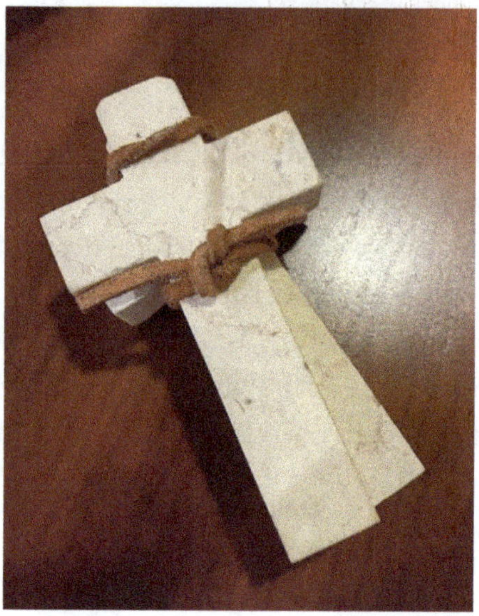

Stone cross that my friend Johnette gave me

Most of all, I remember the nurse who gave me the Xanax. That small act of care became its own kind of lifeline, just enough to calm the storm, let me sleep, and wake up the following morning with some hope of getting through this turmoil.

Those twelve days were a crucible. They tested not just my body, but my spirit. Healing, I learned, is not linear. It is messy, painful, and unpredictable. But it is also filled with moments of grace: people showing up, and strength appearing from nowhere when you need it most.

CHAPTER 5

The Birth of The Shower Shirt™

The first time I was finally able to get out of bed after my bilateral mastectomy, I realized just how dramatically my body had changed. I felt weak, stitched together, and disoriented, as if I were navigating a version of myself I no longer recognized. My movements were slow and deliberate, each one requiring focus and effort. Nothing felt natural anymore.

Then I noticed something else.

Long, transparent plastic drain tubes were sutured into my armpits and hanging all the way down to my knees. At first, my brain struggled to process what I was seeing. I knew my surgeon had mentioned drains, but nothing had prepared me for the reality of four of them, two on each side, each more than four feet long, dangling from my body. They tugged every time I moved, and with each step, I was reminded just how fragile I was. I felt exposed, vulnerable, and profoundly altered.

Within a few days, I was discharged from the hospital with all four drains still in place and given a follow-up appointment for the following morning. When I sat across from my surgeon, whom I call Dr. Z, I asked the most basic and human question imaginable.

"When can I take a shower?"

I will never forget his response. Without hesitation, he said, *"You cannot take a shower until your surgical drains are removed."*

I blinked, convinced I had misunderstood him. *"How long will that be?"*

"Anywhere between two and three weeks," he replied calmly.

I could not believe what I was hearing. I had just undergone a double mastectomy. I smelled like a hospital. My hair was greasy. My chest was covered in blood-stained bandages. I was in pain, emotionally and physically exhausted, and now I was being told I could not even shower.

Dr. Z explained that the drain sites could not get wet because the tubes sutured into my armpits were a direct portal into the surgical site. If bacteria from tap water entered where the tubes met my body, it could lead to a surgical site infection, or SSI, which could devastate the reconstruction process entirely.

It was one of those moments where you think: why did no one tell me this beforehand? The practical, day-to-day realities always seem to arrive as a surprise after the fact. Once home, I immediately began searching online for some kind of water-resistant garment or protective covering that would allow me to shower safely while the drains were still in place.

To my complete disbelief, nothing existed.

I widened my search. Still nothing. I then called several friends and acquaintances who had undergone mastectomies themselves. Every single one told me the same thing.

"I used trash bags," one said. *"Plastic wrap with tape,"* another admitted. *"That's all there was,"* someone else confirmed.

So I tried it too. I wrapped myself in a garbage bag, taped it awkwardly around my shoulders, and did my best to keep the water away from my chest. It was ridiculous. The bag clung to me, shifted constantly, and failed to protect anything in any meaningful way. I had surgical drains dangling from my body that I was trying to stuff underneath it. Standing there, I remember thinking that women had been undergoing mastectomy surgery for over seventy years in this country, and a plastic trash bag was still the best option the medical industry could offer.

Then, while struggling in that shower, I heard a voice repeating: *"Create a water-resistant product. Create a water-resistant product."* At the time, I ignored it. Creating anything was the last thing on my mind.

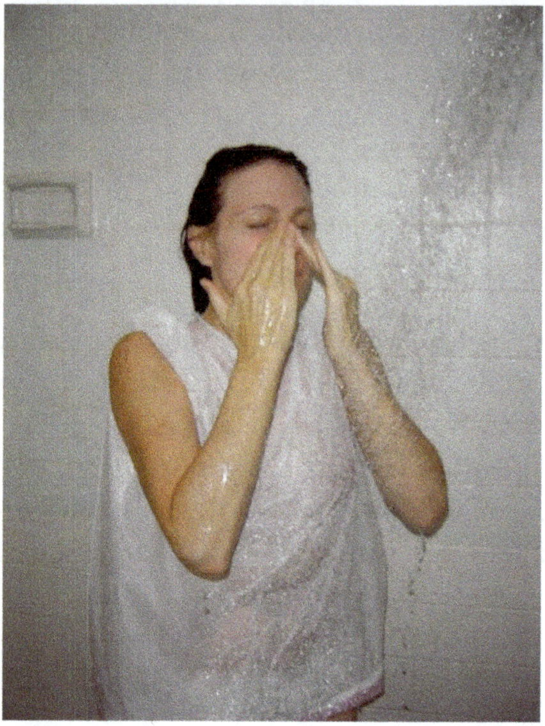

That's Me Showering in a Trash Bag

What made this process more infuriating was that the clinical protocol of keeping surgical drain sites dry existed precisely because of the high infection rates, and the risks and costs associated with those infections in breast cancer related surgeries.

At the time, the American Hospital Association reported that the cost of healthcare tied to surgical site infections following breast cancer surgery was staggering. Studies showed that anywhere from 5% to 29% of patients developed infections. The exact causes were often difficult to determine, but the data included cases linked to waterborne illness.

Even more alarming were the infection rates linked to tissue expander placement, the procedure I had undergone. In some studies, more than 30% of patients developed infections, and of those, 96% were readmitted to the hospital. Nearly every patient with a post-surgical infection found themselves back in a hospital bed.

According to that same AHA study, the median out-of-pocket cost for infected patients was nearly $18,000, compared to $8,000 for uninfected patients. Those figures reflected hospital costs only and did not include physician fees, clinic visits, outpatient procedures, antibiotic intervention, or home health care. And those numbers were from 2010. Today, those costs would be significantly higher.

I did not need statistics to understand the impact. My own hospital bills eventually exceeded $250,000. That alone gives anyone a sense of the financial burden infections can create.

I was part of the 96% of patients who were readmitted, and also part of the 30% who developed infections after tissue expander placement. I understood the fear, the trauma, the emotional toll, and the overwhelming uncertainty that breast cancer patients face.

What I could not understand was why the showering problem had never been addressed. I kept asking myself, and every surgeon I eventually spoke with: is this truly the best the medical industry can offer women after breast cancer surgery?

Especially knowing that showering unprotected, or even in trash bags, can increase the risk of waterborne illness, which in turn increases health risks, clinical complications, and costs.

After developing a serious infection within a week of my initial surgery and enduring the trash bag routine, I became relentless in my search for a solution. I reached out to a close friend and former colleague of more than two decades, Dr. Emran Imami, a breast surgeon I call Dr. E. He was direct and unequivocal.

"Lisa," he said, *"it's quite simple. What comes out of the shower is not sterile. Tap water is loaded with bacteria, parasites, and pathogens. A water-resistant product would be quite helpful for chest surgery patients. By simply taking precautions while showering, you can mitigate waterborne infections and decrease the chances of complications during reconstruction. Infections can be devastating to the reconstruction process."*

Dr. E was such a close friend that I had not sought his services for my mastectomy surgery; we were simply too close for a surgeon-patient relationship. But once I developed an infection and subsequent complications, I sought him out immediately. I genuinely believe he is the reason I have two breasts today, and I will explain why later.

What remained undeniable was the absurd reality that no protective showering garments existed for breast cancer or mastectomy patients. I often joked that if you were a dog who needed a bath, there were dozens of products online designed to make that process easier. But if you were a woman recovering from breast cancer surgery, you were expected to go to your kitchen pantry and grab a trash bag.

From a healthcare standpoint, more than 300,000 women in the United States are diagnosed with breast cancer each year, with nearly 40% undergoing mastectomy surgery. That means more than 100,000 women could benefit from a water-resistant garment designed to protect their surgical drain sites post-surgery.

Being the feminist that I am, I was deeply insulted. That frustration transformed itself into something else entirely. It became a mission, a personal determination, and a drive to make a real difference for patients. I was so incensed by what I had experienced that I did not want one additional patient to feel the way I did.

And yet, I quickly recognized something painfully ironic. Even though I loathed that trash bag, I also depended on it. It became a strange love-hate relationship. By that point, I had been discharged from the hospital twice, once after my mastectomy and again after the infection, both times going home with surgical drains still in place. I had endured the trash bag routine at least a dozen times.

Somewhere in that contradiction, between necessity and outrage, between survival and dignity, the idea began to form. What started as frustration became purpose. What began as indignation turned into innovation.

That was the moment The Shower Shirt™ was born.

I hung that used trash bag in the shower and kept using it day after day while the drains were still in place. To this day, I'm not sure why I never replaced it with a fresh one, but I didn't. That same wrinkled, slightly torn piece of plastic stayed right where it was, hanging over the towel bar.

Somehow, it became my friend. It protected me, sort of. Not well. Not properly. But enough to make me feel safer than standing there completely exposed. It was like having a fair-weather friend: not someone you would trust in a crisis, but someone who shows up just enough to help you get through the moment. After I showered, I felt better physically, and when I felt better physically, I felt better emotionally. At that point in my life, that mattered more than I could explain.

That strange attachment fueled my mission. I kept thinking that if a trash bag could do that for me, even haphazardly, imagine what a proper product, meticulously designed, could do. If I could create a garment that was protective and functionally effective, one that repelled water away from the chest and had internal pockets to support the drains, others might feel that same sense of comfort and safety. My creation could help patients feel better physically, which would help them feel better emotionally and psychologically. I wanted future breast cancer patients to shower without fear. I wanted this garment to become their friend, just as that flimsy trash bag had become mine.

That is when I started sketching. I sat at my kitchen table and drew ideas on napkins, scraps of paper, envelopes, anything I could find. I sent my drawings to my younger brother Charles, an architectural engineer, and asked him to turn my rough ideas into a proper schematic. His first response was, *"What the hell am I supposed to do with this?"*

Simultaneously, my Aunt Marianne and my cousin Mandy got to work on the very first prototype. They took my clumsy sketch and spread it out on the table, studying it like a real blueprint. Using nothing more than a water-resistant beauty salon cape and a lot of determination, they began cutting, pinning, and reshaping the material, slowly turning that rough idea into something we could actually hold in our hands.

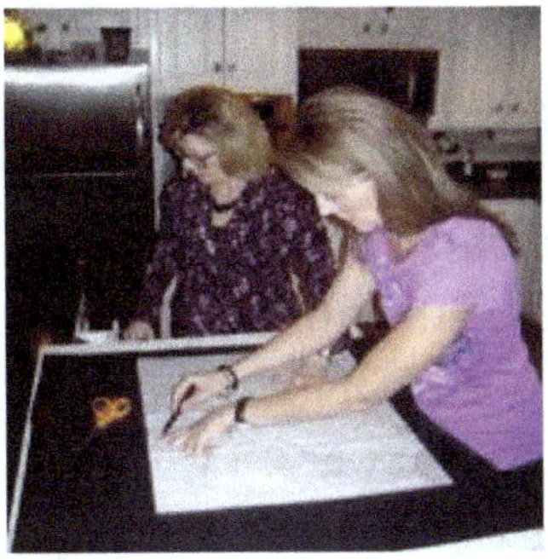

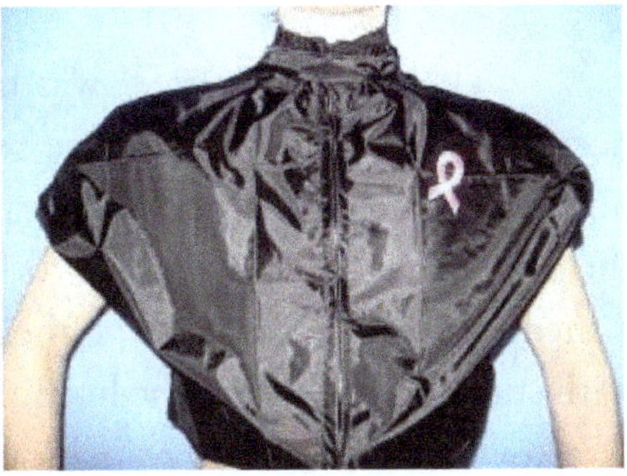

Photos of Aunt Marianne and Mandy working on The Shower Shirt™ prototype.

Once that prototype was finalized, my brother completed the schematic which would eventually become The Shower Shirt™, incorporating water-resistant parachute material, elastic perimeters, cinch straps, work flaps, drain tube straps, and internal pockets designed to hold the drains securely inside.

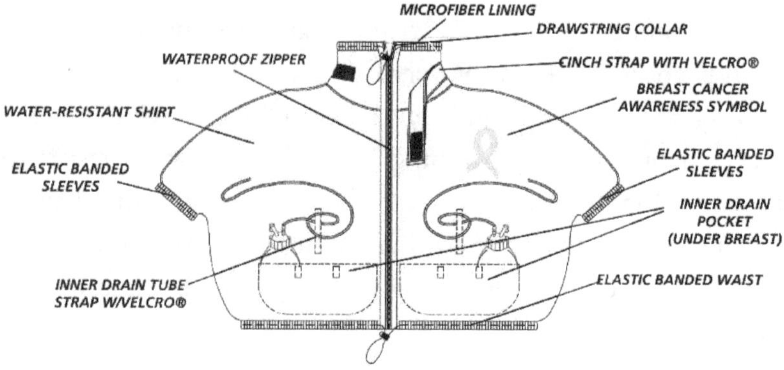

The Shower Shirt™ was born out of frustration and necessity, but it quickly became something much greater: an object with the potential to change patients' lives. I began taking the prototype to doctors I had worked with during my years as a medical reporter, asking for their honest opinions. I spoke with surgeons on staff at the hospital system where I worked as director of media strategy, including Dr. E, who had already become a steadfast supporter of the idea. Every clinician I spoke with responded positively to the drawings, the concepts, and eventually the prototype itself.

The response was consistent.

"Yes, a product like this is highly needed," they told me. *"And not just for breast cancer patients."*

Repeatedly, I heard that this garment could benefit many chest surgery populations who required surgical drains, chemotherapy ports, or catheters for a wide range of medical reasons.

One general surgeon, Dr. Lane, took it even further. He looked at me and said, *"Forget the breast cancer patients. There is a much larger market for the end stage renal disease population."*

He was referring to patients with kidney disease or kidney failure who rely on hemodialysis or peritoneal catheters.

I was not about to forget breast cancer patients. That was my personal connection to this project. That was my *"why."* But what Dr. Lane said opened my eyes to the many other patient populations who could benefit from a protective showering garment.

I began studying kidney disease and quickly learned why those patients also needed showering protection. Through the National Kidney Foundation, I discovered that nearly 100% of end stage renal disease patients eventually acquire infections from catheters, and one of those causes led directly back to waterborne illness, exactly as my surgeon had warned me about.

The clinical threat for those patients is severe. Hemodialysis catheters are typically sutured just above the collarbone, and if an infection occurs, it can enter the bloodstream rapidly and become life-threatening.

Because of my long-standing relationships with several surgeons, I put together a small informal medical advisory board and interviewed each of them about the range of patient populations who could benefit from a protective showering garment. My background in journalism and media strategy became invaluable. I spent months researching every patient population I could identify that relied on chest catheters, ports, or surgical drains.

I studied populations ranging from abdominal hernia surgery patients to cardiac patients requiring pacemaker battery replacements. I learned about patients using wound vacs and infusion pumps, and why their equipment needed protection from water. I found that patients with central lines were highly susceptible to surgical site infections, as were lung surgery and cardiothoracic patients. Rotator cuff patients needed shoulder protection. Bariatric surgery patients required chest coverage. External defibrillator patients, neurostimulation patients, and life vest patients all depended on delicate technology that simply could not get wet.

I kept asking myself the same question. How and why does a protective showering garment not already exist for these patients?

When I asked surgeons directly, they all agreed.

"Nobody has taken the interest that you have," they told me. *"Nobody has tried to create a product specifically to support post-surgical recovery when it comes to showering."*

I shared my idea with another close friend, Jim Lewis. By then, I had shown the prototype to countless doctors, surgeons, and clinicians in my effort to validate the concept. I told Jim I needed a manufacturer who could help me build a second prototype based on the mounting clinical feedback. He suggested I speak with a friend of his named Mike, who worked as an importer of antique car parts from China.

I remember thinking: how could a car parts importer possibly help me?

But he did. He was phenomenal. Mike helped get the entire Shower Shirt manufacturing process off the ground, and before long, I was sending my beauty-salon-inspired prototype to a garment manufacturer in China for review. Within a few weeks, I had several dozen prototypes sitting on my desk.

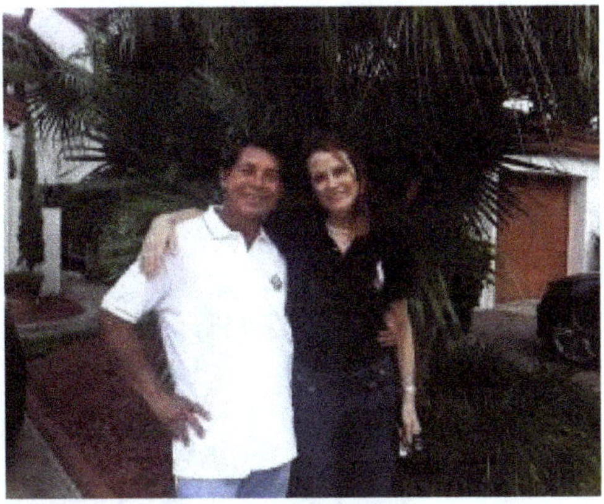

That's Me with Mike Wilson, My Chinese liaison (as I called him)

So, what did I do next? I went back to every surgeon I had spoken with and asked them to give the prototypes to their patients. I needed real feedback from real patients going through surgery and reconstruction. I wanted to know what worked, what didn't, and what needed to change.

I essentially became my own research and development department. Doctors donated The Shower Shirt™ prototypes to their patients, who evaluated them during recovery. And since I was still in and out of the hospital myself due to another infection and additional surgeries, I was using a prototype right alongside them.

Before each procedure, Dr. Z would look at me and say, *"Lisa, remember, you are going to have drains in place, and you need to protect them from water."*

And every time, I would respond, *"Yes, this is not my first rodeo. I have several prototypes to test, so I will be protected."*

For the first time since my diagnosis, I felt like I was no longer just reacting to what was happening to me and my body. I was building something positive. I was reclaiming control of my life.

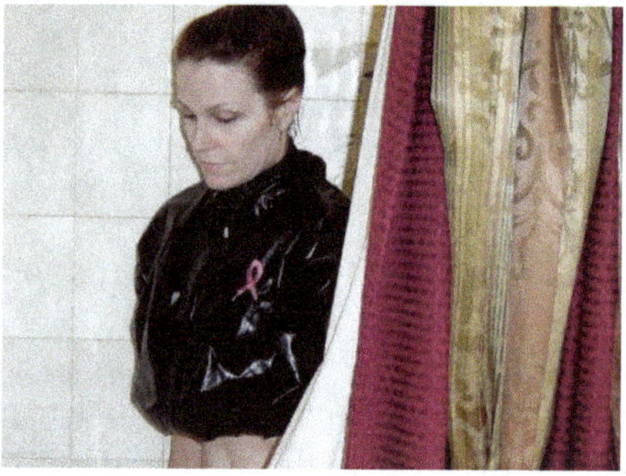

Me testing a Shower Shirt™ prototype

CHAPTER 6

When Pain Meets Purpose

One of my favorite stories to tell from this journey is about a woman named Shannon.

Shannon was a firefighter, strong and fearless, and she had been using one of The Shower Shirt™ prototypes during her recovery. At that time, the early versions of the garment had blocks of Velcro down the front and back work flaps, overlapping panels designed to protect the shirt from water intrusion. The design worked. There had been no water leaks. Clinically, it did exactly what it was supposed to do.

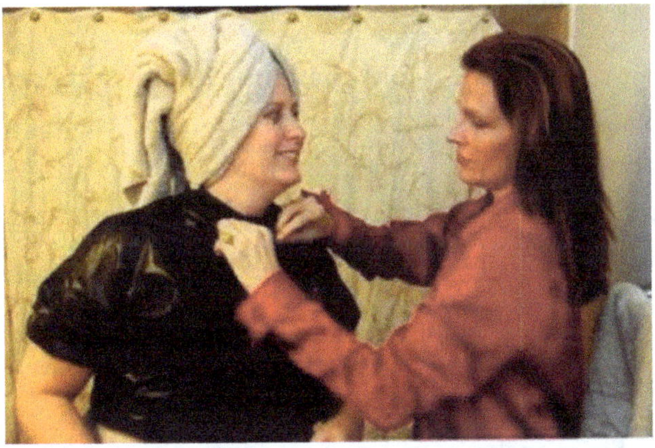

Shannon the Firefighter from a Media feature in Florida Today ® Newspaper.

But Shannon saw something more.

She called me one day and asked if we could meet. When we sat down together, she brought her firefighter jacket and laid it out in front of me. Running straight down the front was one long, wide strip of Velcro®.

She looked at me and said, *"This is what protects me when I run into burning buildings."*

Then she suggested I update The Shower Shirt™ with that same elongated Velcro design. It was a brilliant idea. Even though she had experienced no water intrusion with the original prototype, her suggestion added an extra layer of protection, security, and confidence. It was practical. It was intuitive. It came from someone whose life depended on protective gear. That moment reinforced something I was already learning: the best innovations come from listening to the people who actually use the product.

After countless conversations with breast cancer surgery patients who had become part of my informal research and development team, I met again with Mike to make further updates. In total, we went through five prototypes before deciding we were ready to go to market.

While all of this was happening, my body was still in uncertain and somewhat disorderly crisis.

Six months later, I was readmitted to the hospital. My surgeon needed to insert a new left tissue expander, as the first had been removed due to the initial MRSA infection. Once the second expander was inserted, I came down with yet another infection. Seven days after my third surgery, following the initial mastectomy, the removal of the first tissue expander, and the insertion of another, I found myself once again facing the possibility of bodily disaster.

I had an appointment with Dr. Z at four o'clock that afternoon. I told him I was not feeling well and that I was concerned I might have another infection. It had been seven days since my last surgery, the same timeframe in which my first infection had surfaced six months earlier, so I was nervous.

Without hesitation, he said, *"Lisa, there is no reason for me to believe you have an infection. But if you don't feel well in the middle of the night, call your primary physician."*

I had heard those exact words before. The first time was when I called him in the middle of the night with that initial infection.

I was stunned.

It was an insensitive response, but I was emotional and scared. I feared another infection. I feared losing the option to reconstruct my breasts. I feared another surgery. Still, I did not push back. I did not argue. I did not even respond with sarcasm.

I wasn't myself.

I had slipped back into the little girl who once feared her father, and now feared this surgeon. I depended on him to keep me alive, to keep me healthy, to keep me uninfected. So I simply said, *"Okay."*

Sure enough, in the middle of the night, I became sick again. I could barely hold my head up, and back to the emergency department I went, with infection draining from my post-surgical drain.

I knew then that it was time to change surgeons. He was skilled, with unwavering credentials, but his poor bedside manner and lack of empathy were no longer something I could ignore. The problem was that I was considered a complicated patient, and I knew no other surgeon would take me on. Surgeons run from infections. They run from patients with a history of complications. I had to stick with Dr. Z and keep my mouth shut, sarcasm firmly under control.

Despite fearing most everything at that point, there was one thing I did not fear.

I did not fear creating a water-resistant garment for breast cancer patients, if I could just stay healthy enough to stay on course. What I felt was becoming my calling kept me alive in ways medicine could not. It anchored me during the mental and physical distress that threatened to overpower me.

Six months earlier, during the first infection, the infectious disease doctor had shared his concern that the MRSA was hospital acquired. He had initially believed I was infected during surgery with an unsterile tissue expander, and when the infection returned, it felt like confirmation of exactly what he had feared.

This infection was also MRSA.

He explained that when MRSA embeds itself into the skin, or the chest wall in this case, it can go dormant under high doses of antibiotic therapy. With the chest wall having been opened again through a surgical incision, the infection had resurfaced. *"This is a recurrence of the same MRSA infection,"* he said, *"which has been dormant for a few months."*

Fortunately, the second infection was not nearly as advanced as the first. I had known something was off the day before, when I was in Dr. Z's office, even though he hadn't caught it. I am grateful I trusted my instincts and returned to the hospital the moment my temperature spiked.

After this second infection, I began studying hospital infection rates associated with MRSA. According to the Centers for Disease Control and Prevention, MRSA accounts for roughly 10% of all hospital-associated infections in the United States. I was disheartened to find myself part of that statistic. MRSA is resistant to typical antibiotic therapies, something I have had to manage carefully over the years, and will address in later chapters.

I also began reading about hyperbaric oxygen therapy, or HBOT, for severe wound infections including MRSA. HBOT enhances the body's natural healing process by having the patient breathe 100% pure oxygen in a pressurized chamber, increasing oxygen levels in blood plasma ten to twenty times higher than normal. It is widely used to treat chronic wounds, severe infections, and radiation injuries, and is also well known for helping divers who develop decompression sickness. I wondered if I might be a candidate.

I asked Dr. Z about it.

He dismissed it immediately. *"That's goobledy-gosh,"* he said.

To this day, I am not sure what that term means. Regardless, the idea was brushed aside.

So, I did what I had done for nearly two decades. I reached out to my trusted friend and clinical advisor, Dr. E.

As it turned out, Dr. E was the medical director of a hospital-based hyperbaric oxygen therapy facility connected to the very same hospital system where I was employed.

He did not hesitate.

"Lisa," he said, *"you would be a perfect candidate for this type of intensive wound care treatment."*

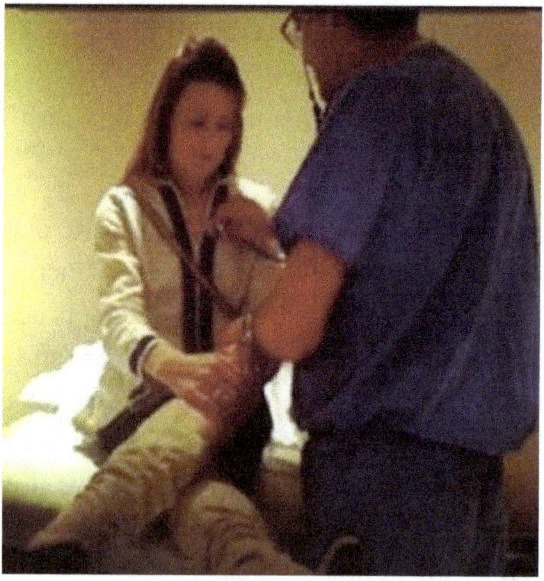

Dr. Emran Imami checking my vitals before Hyperbaric Oxygen Treatments

Within a few days and multiple rounds of antibiotics, I was discharged from the hospital with a PICC line, a peripherally inserted catheter sutured into my right arm, connected to an IV stand carrying a bag of Vancomycin, the antibiotic used for systemic MRSA infections. Post-surgical drains were still hanging from my left armpit. The PICC line was required because Vancomycin could not be pushed through a smaller IV due to an increased risk of scar tissue in the veins. The surgical drains remained in place so doctors could monitor the discharge of infection. I looked like a walking clinical freakshow, with appendages connected to both sides of me and a steel contraption trailing behind me wherever I went.

Because of these complications, my surgeon ordered daily visits from home health nurses for the first seven days. Their job was twofold: to ensure there were no issues with the PICC line, which was yet another potential source of infection, and to closely monitor the output from the surgical drains to confirm the Vancomycin was bringing the second infection under control. The longer the drains remained in place, however, the higher the risk of another infection. It was a constant balancing act requiring vigilance and patience.

Before this latest infection, and before my third hospital admission in just six months, I had been actively testing The Shower Shirt™ designs and tailoring them to different patient populations. Ironically, just before my discharge, a nurse casually instructed me to wrap the PICC line in plastic and tape it before showering, since the catheter could not get wet.

I almost laughed.

PICC line patients were yet another group who needed The Shower Shirt™.

The nurse went on to explain the risks of bacteria and pathogens in tap water, reminding me that because the catheter was sutured directly into my arm, the area had to remain completely dry to prevent a waterborne infection. I wanted to shout it from the roof: I'm building something for PICC line patients too! Instead, I smiled quietly and thought to myself that maybe God was guiding me exactly where I needed to go. My job was simply to listen, learn, and keep moving forward.

I often wondered whether enduring that second infection had a purpose beyond my own healing, to introduce me to yet another patient population that could benefit from a protective garment. After all, an estimated three million PICC lines are placed in patients every year in the United States alone. With that realization came a change in design: the sleeves needed to be longer to fully protect PICC line patients.

Seven days later, I returned to Dr. Z's office, where the surgical drain was finally removed. The infection output had decreased, proof that the Vancomycin was working and the MRSA was receding. I felt immediate relief. With the drains gone, I could prepare to begin HBOT treatments without the burden of managing yet another medical appendage inside the chamber.

Dr. E wasted no time. Within a week, IV stand in tow, I found myself at the hyperbaric oxygen therapy center, being fitted with headgear that looked like something an astronaut might wear, along with hospital scrubs and monitoring equipment.

I spent five hours a day, four days a week, inside that chamber. The HBOT team was extraordinary. They became family. Each of them understood that every patient entering that chamber was fighting an unseen enemy, whether infection, cancer, limb loss, chronic wounds, or another serious condition. They were kind, patient, and deeply empathetic, everything a healthcare provider needs to be when a patient is at their most vulnerable.

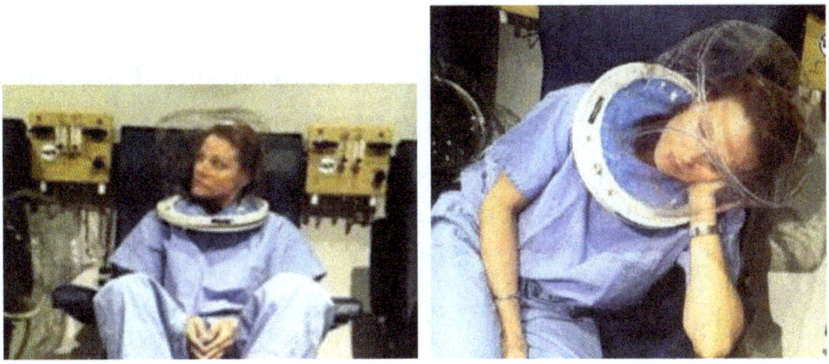

That's me in the Hyperbaric Oxygen Treatment Chamber

Through all of it, The Shower Shirt™ mission continued to evolve, and every setback pushed me forward. Each morning, it was the first thought in my mind. Each night, it was the last. Every afternoon when I left the hyperbaric chamber, I would go home and think about how to move the project forward. Every infection, every surgery, every doctor visit, every time I looked down and saw drains hanging from my body, I reminded myself that one day, women would have an easier recovery because of what I was building.

The Shower Shirt™ became my purpose, my focus, the project that kept me sane and grounded when every other part of my life felt uncertain. Even in my lowest moments, and especially during those HBOT treatments, I felt my mother's presence urging me forward. She had always devoted herself to meaningful work through her philanthropic efforts, and in some ways, she was still guiding me, helping me turn my pain into purpose. I knew she would have been thrilled by this.

I began reading a book called *Unstoppable: Powerful Stories of Perseverance and Triumph* by Cynthia Kersey. It chronicled the journeys of companies that had struggled deeply, some facing bankruptcy, before ultimately achieving massive success, including brands like Disney and Domino's Pizza. One passage stopped me in my tracks. The author wrote that it is harder to bring a product to market that has never existed than to take an existing product, change it by five to ten percent, and rebrand it.

That line felt like it had been written directly for me.

I was attempting the harder path. I was trying to bring a product to market that had never existed before. I knew it would be a difficult fight, but by that point I was ready, as long as I could stay healthy and out of the hospital long enough to see it through.

For the first time since my diagnosis, I felt in control again. And that made every ounce of the pain worth it.

CHAPTER 7

Where Fear Meets Conviction

Eventually, after months of listening to patients, studying their feedback, and refining the prototypes, including the adjustments for PICC line patients, I knew it was time. The Shower Shirt™ was ready for its first real order. Through Mike, my manufacturing liaison, I learned that the factory required a minimum run of 700 shirts. By then, money was moving out faster than it was coming in. Patent research had already begun, savings were thinning, and every decision carried weight. Still, I placed the order.

That moment was terrifying.

When the wire transfer was finally sent, I sat there and thought: even if this entire mission fails, I will be okay. All I wanted was to sell one Shower Shirt to one patient. If I could help even a single person shower safely and with dignity, then the financial sweat and tears poured into creating this product would have been worth it. Of course, I dreamed of helping hundreds of thousands. But I had made peace with the idea that helping just one would be enough. Even if 699 shirts sat untouched in boxes, at least one person would have benefited, and that alone would make me proud.

The doctors on my medical advisory board each asked if they could invest. Their confidence meant more to me than the money itself. Still, I was not ready to give up creative control or the months of work I had already poured into the project. I thanked them sincerely and chose instead to keep dipping into my own savings.

That decision was not easy. Ongoing breast cancer complications had forced me onto short-term disability, and I could no longer work full time. Every dollar mattered. Pouring money into this labor of love was financially exhausting, but emotionally, it felt necessary.

Before this journey began, I had always been one of those proudly loyal Americans who questioned why so many products were manufactured outside the United States. I wanted this garment produced at home. I tried. When Mike and I first spoke, I made that preference clear. He worked his contacts, but the numbers came back impossible. Manufacturing in the US would cost $73 per shirt, making the final retail price unaffordable for most patients. I had set a target retail price of $78 to keep it accessible, so that reality forced a difficult decision, and manufacturing moved overseas.

Over the years, I continued searching for alternatives, meeting with respected companies in Portugal, Mexico, India, Turkey, Costa Rica, and additional US-based facilities. Time and again, the result was the same. None could match the balance of quality and cost we had already secured.

While production plans moved forward, I began the formal process of protecting what we had created. I was introduced to Christopher Brody, a patent attorney in the Washington, D.C. area who had spent eight years as a patent examiner with the United States Patent and Trademark Office.

That background gave me confidence. I shared my vision, the architectural drawings my brother had created, and the most recent prototype.

After extensive research, he confirmed what I had quietly hoped. There was nothing like it. While protective products existed, such as plastic coverings, foot sleeves, and flat barriers, no one had created a garment specifically designed to protect the chest during showering.

As the patent process unfolded, I did as much of the work myself as I could to manage costs. I wrote portions of the application, formed an LLC, and named it The Shower Shirt Co. I collaborated with graphic designers on branding, created a logo, and began imagining what the website might look like. I also started talking to people inside hospitals, home medical equipment providers, durable medical equipment suppliers, and hospital gift shops, sharing this simple idea born from personal necessity.

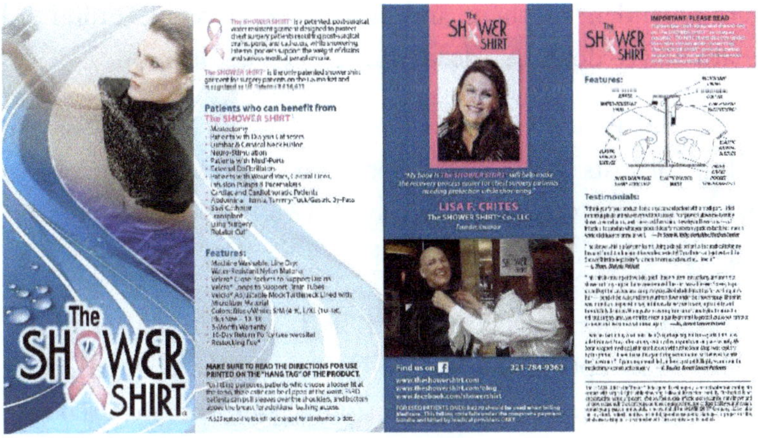

To my surprise, after only a handful of meetings, I received a purchase order from a hospital system for 500 shirts. Just like that, I had blown past my original goal. I did not sell just one Shower Shirt. I sold another 499 right behind it.

I was thrilled. And then reality set in.

I had only ordered 700 shirts. That meant I would have just 200 left once the order shipped. Still, I reminded myself this was a good problem to have. I would recoup a portion of my investment quickly, and I desperately needed those funds to cover the mounting patent costs.

With the initial order nearly depleted, it was time to place a second. When I called Mike, the news was distressing. The manufacturer had increased the minimum order quantity to 2,000 units. That single change nearly bankrupted the company. The original agreement had been 700 units, and the number had nearly tripled overnight, taking the investment from roughly $20,000 to $60,000. The manufacturer knew we were dependent on them, and I had no real leverage. Still, I did what I had to do: take a deep breath and wire the money.

Fortunately, Mike agreed to cover a portion of the additional costs until I could repay him. The lesson I took from that experience was simple: always have a Plan B manufacturer when bringing a product to market.

Not long after, we did find another manufacturer willing to accept smaller orders. Unfortunately, they struggled to work with the heavy, water-resistant parachute material that made The Shower Shirt™ what it was. Seams failed.

Production suffered. After just one order, that relationship ended.

The third time was the charm.

We found MEELYNN Garment Company, and they would go on to become trusted partners for more than a decade. Their team specialized in producing luxury blouses for the European fashion market. When I saw their work, I thought: if they can create garments selling for nearly 400 euros, they can certainly produce a durable, water-resistant shirt. They proved me right.

While manufacturing transitions unfolded, the patent process continued in parallel. We filed a provisional patent application, which granted us temporary patent pending status. Exactly one year later, the application was denied.

Mr. Brody called to explain that the USPTO believed we were infringing on several existing patents. He sent me the list of citations, and I went to work. For nearly two weeks, I reviewed every reference line by line, writing detailed responses explaining why The Shower Shirt™ did not infringe on any existing intellectual property. None of the cited patents resembled our design or method of use. The majority had never even been brought to market.

I was frustrated. How could they claim infringement on something that did not exist, either commercially or in practice? If it had existed, thousands of mastectomy patients, including me, would not have been reduced to showering with trash bags taped to their bodies.

I later learned that rejection is not the exception at the USPTO. It is the rule. Nearly 90% of patent applications are initially denied, and roughly 70% of those are eventually approved after amendments and persistence. The process is designed to test resolve.

My patent attorney quickly learned two things about me. I was determined, and I was impatient. He laughed often and reminded me to slow down. But I did not have the luxury of time. Five hundred shirts were already sold and in transit, and I needed protection immediately. He reassured me that once the second application was filed, we would again have patent-pending status. Then he said something I will never forget: *"Lisa, you go out and market your ass off. Let me worry about the patent."*

So, I did.

We submitted the amended application, paying for the process all over again. Then, just three weeks later, the impossible happened. We were granted an official United States patent. I memorized the number instantly.

I remember the call clearly. Mr. Brody said, *"Lisa, this is your lucky day."* He spoke slowly, with a soft Southern drawl. I interrupted him and said, *"Mr. Brody, you are too expensive to talk this slowly. Please speed it up."* He laughed, then explained that The Shower Shirt™ had been awarded a patent not only for its design, but also for its method of use. That combination, he told me, was considered the gold standard in patent protection. I felt extremely blessed, and honored, especially after learning that only 7% of women in the United States (at the time) held patents, with the other 93% awarded to men.

With our intellectual property finally secure, I felt a calm I had not known in months. I was ready to market my ass off.

Not long after, a friend who managed a hospital gift shop within the same healthcare system where I worked told me I needed to join Essentially Women, a US-based group purchasing organization serving hospital gift shops, home health companies, and mastectomy boutiques. I researched it immediately and joined. It was another significant investment, but by then I understood that investment was simply part of momentum.

With patent protection in place, I began speaking with medical device distribution companies interested in representing the product. I also wanted an experienced partner to present alongside me at my first conference. Several companies showed immediate interest, particularly after learning we had already sold 500 units. One introduction led me to Tim Crowley, an international distribution representative whose approach and integrity stood out from the start.

After just a few conversations, I knew I wanted to work with his team.

We were headed to Phoenix, Arizona, for our first Essentially Women conference. It felt like the beginning of something much bigger than I had ever imagined.

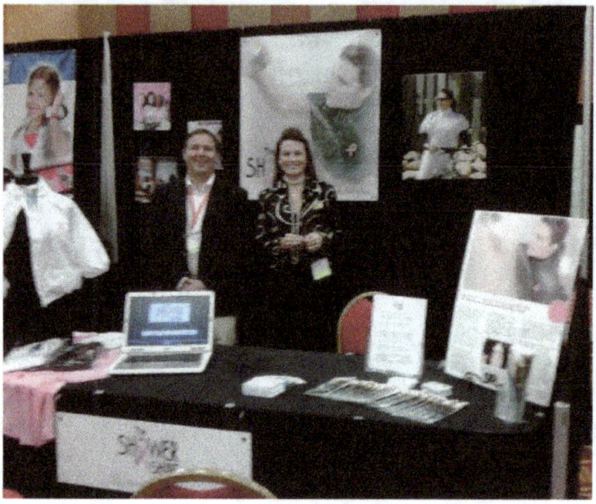

Tim Crowley and Me at the Essentially Women Conference

Essentially Women was the perfect alliance for introducing the product to their extensive client base. Through their conference promotions, buyers knew who we were before we had a chance to know them.

If I am perfectly honest, that conference was just as validating as receiving the patent. Every single day, clinicians stopped at the booth and confirmed what I had felt all along. The need was real. I heard it repeatedly. People told me they had come to the conference specifically to see The Shower Shirt™.

Nurses, surgeons, breast navigators, social workers, dialysis clinic representatives, mastectomy boutique owners, and buyers from home medical and durable medical equipment companies came from all over the country. Person after person said the same thing: *"We've been dealing with mastectomy patients for years without an appropriate product to shower in. I wanted to see this for myself."*

For three straight days, there was a line at The Shower Shirt™ booth. It was exhilarating. It was also overwhelming.

My health was still fragile. I had additional surgeries ahead of me as part of the reconstruction process, and I was still emotionally managing the reality of having only one breast and one tissue expander. I was still afraid that another infection would surface when they eventually swapped the expander for the final implant. But that weekend carried me in a way I had not expected. It became a powerful part of my healing, at least mentally and psychologically.

It was also the first time I truly paused to consider what I was building. Until then, I had focused almost entirely on the risks: the money I could lose, the reasons it might fail, the very real possibility that this could all collapse. But standing there, watching clinicians' line up to talk about a product I had created, a new question surfaced. What if this actually works? And quietly behind it: what comes next?

That thought unsettled me.

I was not a businessperson. I was a medical journalist on a corporate media hiatus. I was not a seasoned inventor. I was an accidental one. I never set out to become an entrepreneur, and yet there I was, stepping into the healthcare industry from an entirely new angle, no longer as a journalist or a hospital-based media strategist, but as the owner of a home health medical product. Even with all the excitement and validation, I felt the weight of that shift.

During the conference, Tim Crowley and I spent a great deal of time discussing the need for a dedicated HCPCS code for The Shower Shirt™. HCPCS, the Healthcare Common Procedure Coding System, is a standardized billing code maintained by the Centers for Medicare and Medicaid Services and used by insurers nationwide. Without one, the product could not be reimbursed through insurance.

That, it became clear, was the next mountain.

Nearly every buyer who visited the booth asked the same question: Does it have an individual HCPCS code? Each time, I was reminded of what I had read in *"Unstoppable"*: it is far more difficult to bring a product to market that has never existed than to modify something that already does. Because nothing comparable to The Shower Shirt™ had ever been created, we would have to start from the very beginning with the government to obtain a proper medical billing classification. I had no idea how vast and complicated that process would become. I would learn soon enough.

That conference changed everything. It put the company on the map. Orders began coming in steadily. Dialysis centers started calling, just as Dr. Lane had predicted, confirming a significant unmet need in that patient population as well.

While we initiated the HCPCS application process, The Shower Shirt™ remained a self-pay item, which slowed early growth. But it was available. Women finally had an option other than a trash bag, and that had always been the heart of the mission.

That weekend marked the moment when an idea born from personal necessity became something much larger. It became proof that dignity still had a place in healthcare.

CHAPTER 8

Blind Faith

The Shower Shirt™ journey began in June 2009, just four weeks after my double mastectomy. My body was still healing, my energy was limited, and emotionally, I was still trying to make sense of everything that had happened. Still, I had a clear and almost unthinkable goal: I wanted this product on the market by October 2010.

It was ambitious, and I knew it. But I had my heart set on October because October is Breast Cancer Awareness Month. If this product was ever going to matter, if it was ever going to reach the women who truly needed it, that was the moment. I wanted at least one company to agree to carry it and begin selling it that month. Just one. That felt like enough.

What followed was a year of constant refinement. Five evolving prototypes. Dozens of breast cancer patients willing to evaluate them. Conversations that began with vulnerability and ended with honest feedback. We adjusted seams, closures, fit, and fabric over and over again. Every change was driven by authentic experience, including my own. I tested every version myself, because I knew exactly what it felt like to stand in a bathroom wanting nothing more than a safe, normal shower.

Once we had placed the first manufacturing order and a hospital system had placed a 500-unit order within weeks of it, I knew we could meet the deadline. That order became the turning point. It was the moment we could finally say that The

Shower Shirt™ had entered the market during Breast Cancer Awareness Month, just as I had hoped.

The October rollout was intentional. Years before cancer entered my life, I had worked as a news reporter. I understood how editors and producers thought, especially during awareness months when they were actively searching for meaningful, human-centered stories. I also understood the narrative. A former health and medical television reporter turned breast cancer survivor, who invented a product for patients like herself, was a story that made sense. We were ready to share it.

We sent out one press release.

That was all it took.

One of the first invitations came from Lifetime TV's morning show, The Balancing Act. I remember hanging up the phone and thinking: the website isn't even finished. As soon as the call ended, I reached out to the team building The Shower Shirt™ website and told them they had to finish it immediately, because we were going to be on national television.

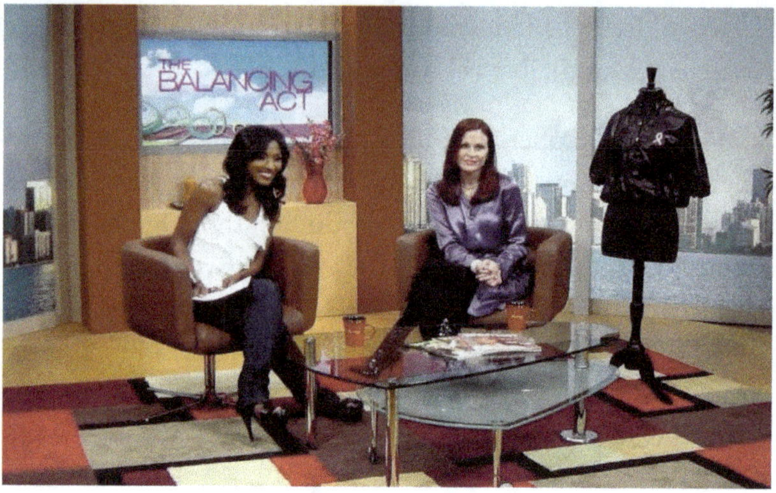

Lifetime TV's 'The Balancing Act' Morning Show

The interview itself was expansive and deeply personal. I shared my breast cancer journey and talked openly about showering with trash bags taped to my chest. I explained how unacceptable that reality was for women already enduring so much. This wasn't about building a business for profit. It was about dignity. It was about giving patients something better.

After the segment aired, everything accelerated. Fox News morning programs invited me to share the story in Orlando, St. Louis, Memphis, Atlanta, and Nashville. Newspapers and magazines started calling. Reporters wanted to understand how something so obvious had never before existed. It all felt surreal. I expected the story to resonate, but I had no idea how far it would travel, or how quickly.

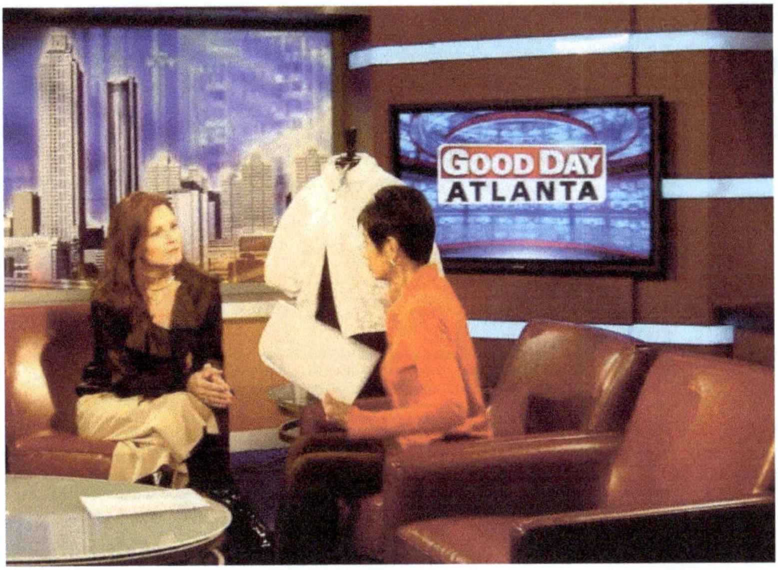

FOX News Good Day Atlanta Morning Show

Essentially Women played a significant role during this period. They promoted every media feature to thousands of healthcare industry members, giving us credibility just as we were entering the market. Joining them had felt like a significant financial risk at the time, but it turned out to be one of the smartest early decisions we made.

The recognition continued to grow. The Shower Shirt™ was featured in the book *Women Inventors and the Top 7-Percent* by Robert Bear. One of my favorite moments came when we were featured in Forbes magazine by medical writer Dr. Elaine Schattner. I often joke that I must be the poorest person ever to appear in Forbes, but none of that mattered. We were there.

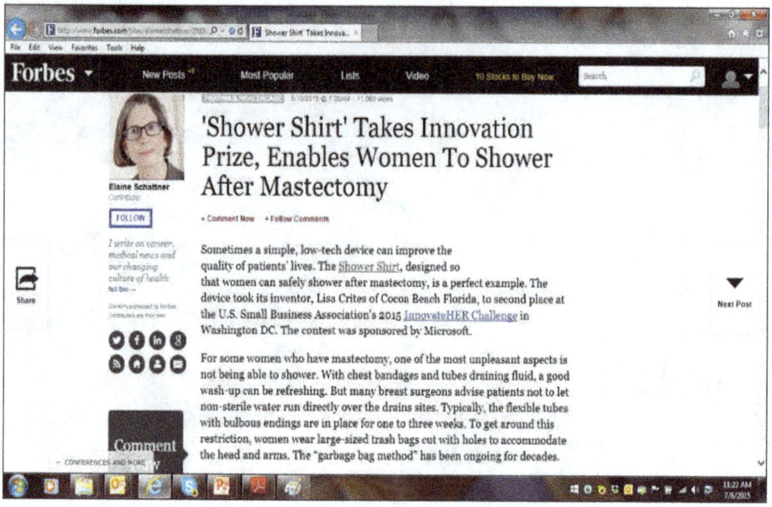

Forbes
New Posts
Most Popular
Lists
Video
10 Stocks to Buy Now

Elaine Schattner

FOLLOW

I write on cancer, medical news and our changing culture of health

'Shower Shirt' Takes Innovation Prize, Enables Women To Shower After Mastectomy

+ Comment Now + Follow Comments

Sometimes a simple, low-tech device can improve the quality of patients' lives. The Shower Shirt, designed so that women can safely shower after mastectomy, is a perfect example. The device took its inventor, Lisa Crites of Cocoa Beach Florida, to second place at the U.S. Small Business Association's 2015 InnovateHER Challenge in Washington DC. The contest was sponsored by Microsoft.

For some women who have mastectomy, one of the most unpleasant aspects is not being able to shower. With chest bandages and tubes draining fluid, a good wash-up can be refreshing. But many breast surgeons advise patients not to let non-sterile water run directly over the drains sites. Typically, the flexible tubes with bulbous endings are in place for one to three weeks. To get around this restriction, women wear large-sized trash bags cut with holes to accommodate the head and arms. The "garbage bag method" has been ongoing for decades.

Forbes Magazine Excerpt

Another feature that meant a great deal to me appeared in the Huffington Post as part of actress and producer Rita Wilson's Voices of Strength series. Rita had also gone through breast cancer and created a space for stories rooted in honesty and resilience. Being included was a genuine honor.

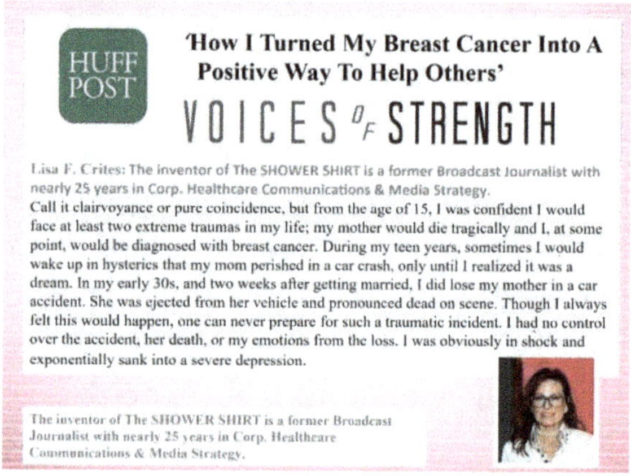

HUFF POST

'How I Turned My Breast Cancer Into A Positive Way To Help Others'

VOICES OF STRENGTH

Lisa F. Crites: The inventor of The SHOWER SHIRT is a former Broadcast Journalist with nearly 25 years in Corp. Healthcare Communications & Media Strategy.

Call it clairvoyance or pure coincidence, but from the age of 15, I was confident I would face at least two extreme traumas in my life; my mother would die tragically and I, at some point, would be diagnosed with breast cancer. During my teen years, sometimes I would wake up in hysterics that my mom perished in a car crash, only until I realized it was a dream. In my early 30s, and two weeks after getting married, I did lose my mother in a car accident. She was ejected from her vehicle and pronounced dead on scene. Though I always felt this would happen, one can never prepare for such a traumatic incident. I had no control over the accident, her death, or my emotions from the loss. I was obviously in shock and exponentially sank into a severe depression.

The inventor of The SHOWER SHIRT is a former Broadcast Journalist with nearly 25 years in Corp. Healthcare Communications & Media Strategy.

Huffington Post "Voices of Strength"

We were also invited to present at the Huffington Post's Entrepreneurs Start-Up exhibition during the 2012 Republican National Convention in Tampa, Florida. The invitation came shortly after a guest column I wrote was published in the Orlando Business Journal, discussing the challenges small businesses face in obtaining Medicare coverage for The Shower Shirt™. The timing was fitting: it was spring 2012, and every politician was campaigning on growing small businesses.

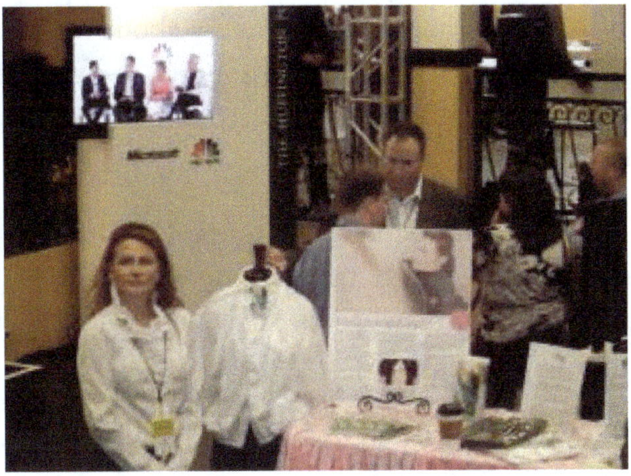

The Shower Shirt™ booth at the Huffington Post Republican National Convention Exhibit

I grew up in a staunchly Democratic family, married two devoted Republicans, and registered as an Independent, so when the opportunity came, I knew I might need to set aside labels. Party politics didn't matter that day. The Huffington Post's focus was clear: connecting innovative start-ups with exposure, support, and networking opportunities.

One moment from that event still makes me smile. A small, energetic team approached my booth, eager to share their idea for a new app. They called their company Uber and explained, almost dreamily, that they hoped one day people would say *"Let's Uber it"* the way they said *"Google it."* At the time, it sounded ambitious. Today, I can't help but grin. They absolutely got their wish.

As media attention grew, something became clear on the consumer side. Unless someone had personally gone through a mastectomy or chest surgery, or supported someone who had, they simply did not know about the no-showering rule. The idea that surgical drains, ports, and catheters sutured into the body, could not be exposed to water was unfamiliar to most people.

That realization mattered. We were not only introducing a product that had never existed; we were also educating people on why it needed to exist in the first place.

Medical professionals understood immediately. Infection prevention and protecting healing sites were second nature to them. But the average person had never encountered that information, and even I hadn't fully understood it before my surgery, despite more than a decade as a medical journalist.

As we began attending breast cancer support conferences and consumer-facing events, this gap came up continuously. People would stop at the booth, point to the image on our display, and ask why the woman in the shower was wearing a shirt. They would usually follow that with: *"Does this have something to do with breast cancer?"*

It does. And so much more.

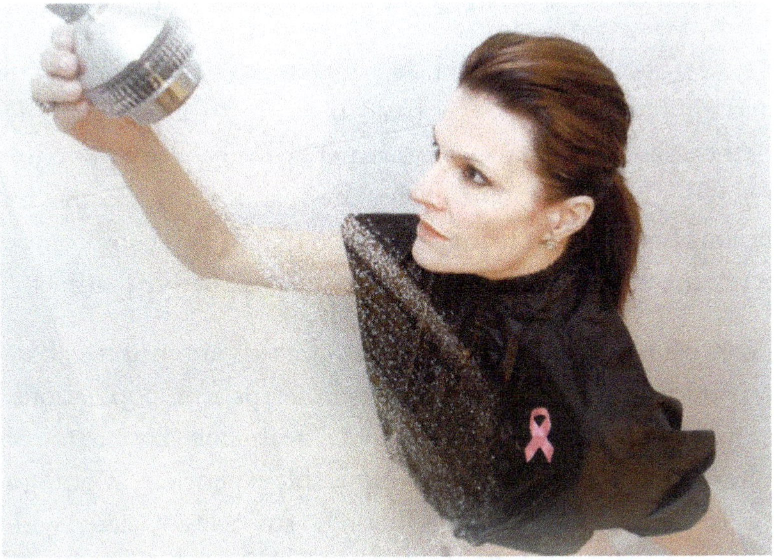

That was why we chose such a simple, self-explanatory image for our branding. It invited curiosity and conversation. The pink ribbon made the connection unmistakable. For decades it had represented hope, support, remembrance, and early detection. It was universally recognized and part of the public domain.

Once we committed to that symbolism, the decision was easy. We embroidered the ribbon directly onto the shirt. It wasn't just branding. It was a statement, a visible acknowledgment of the community this product was created for and the reason it existed.

Over time, we made the decision to remove it. It was not an easy choice, because that ribbon carried deep meaning for me and for the community the product was originally created to serve. But two realities made the decision unavoidable.

The first was practical. The embroidery, as beautiful and symbolic as it was, eventually began to affect the integrity of the water-resistant parachute material. Every needle puncture created a potential point of weakness, and when it comes to healing bodies and infection risk, even the smallest compromise is too much. Protecting patients had to come before sentiment.

The second reason became clear as our customer base expanded. We were now serving other patient populations, especially men undergoing dialysis treatment. For many of them, showering was already a vulnerable experience. Wearing a garment marked with a pink ribbon, so strongly associated with breast cancer, added another layer of difficulty to an already hard moment. What had once been a powerful symbol for one community was unintentionally becoming a barrier for another.

Removing the ribbon did not erase its meaning. It simply allowed the shirt to serve more people with the same dignity it had always been intended to provide.

Once the product entered the market, the first year unfolded in a whirlwind. Growth was steady, and from places I never could have predicted. We expanded to more than forty retail distributors. Walmart's medical device division began carrying the product, which was virtually unheard of for something that had just entered the market. Historically, they only purchased products with at least a five-year retail track record. The American Cancer Society's retail arm, TLC, began shipping it not only across the United States but into Canada and Europe. We partnered with Cure Diva and Health Products For You, an e-commerce platform with more than one million customers. Mastectomy boutiques, medical supply stores, and home medical equipment providers across the country began stocking The Shower Shirt™.

The growth was encouraging, though not as fast as it might have been. We were still facing significant hurdles with government billing and reimbursement. Without the appropriate coding, the product could not be covered by Medicare or most insurance plans, which meant it remained a self-pay item and slowed adoption within large healthcare systems.

Still, we were selling shirts. And to me, that was everything.

Even without regulatory reimbursement, my focus never changed. I wanted a protective garment to exist so women would no longer be forced to shower with tape and plastic. If the product was on the market and available to patients, it had already succeeded in my eyes.

Our team completed The Shower Shirt™ website just in time for our appearance on Lifetime TV's The Balancing Act in early October 2010. Once the site went live, I discovered something I hadn't expected. I loved connecting directly with patients.

Every order felt personal. I knew those shirts were going straight to someone who needed them. Each purchase represented one person being helped, whether bought for personal use or sent as a gift by a friend or family member. Each shirt had a purpose, and each destination mattered.

Over time, I began to think of The Shower Shirt™ customers as a new kind of sisterhood. A club no one ever asked to join, but once inside, you instinctively wanted to help others. These women now knew there was an option. Trash bags were no longer the only option.

To them, I may have been simply the owner of a small company. But to me, they were something much more. They were a constant reminder of where I had been and why this work mattered.

I often say that we never marketed The Shower Shirt™ in the traditional sense. Between Essentially Women sharing the product with their members, media features, and organic word of mouth, we simply put it into the universe. And somehow, it found its way to the people who needed it.

I made it a point to call customers whenever I could, especially those who reached out immediately after surgery. I worried about them. I remembered exactly what it felt like to stand where they were, unable to shower because of drains and fear and uncertainty. That memory never left me.

I also prioritized shipping retail orders within 24 hours whenever possible. That wasn't about customer service metrics. It was instinct. It was one woman taking care of another. It felt protective, personal, and necessary.

For the first time, I truly felt like I was making a difference. One shirt at a time. One patient at a time. That realization gave me a deep sense of happiness and the strength to keep moving forward.

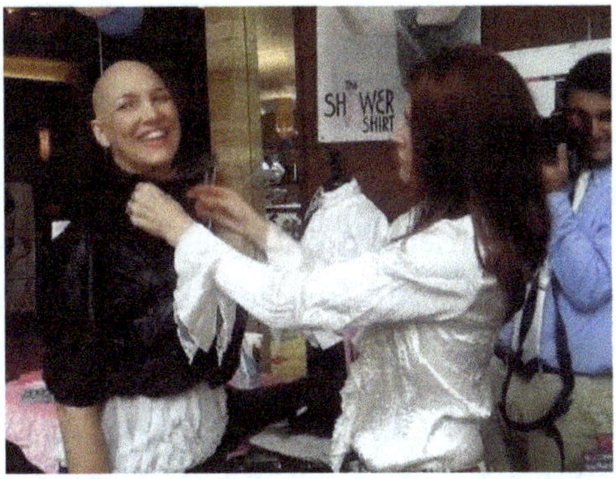

Miami Breast Cancer Conference

It was also the first time I allowed myself to look back. I had been so focused on the next step that I had not stopped to reflect on everything that had transpired over the previous year and a half. So much work and dedication had unfolded in such a short span of time.

Guided by what I can only describe as blind faith, I had prayed more during that period than I ever had in my life. I prayed for my health. I prayed for guidance. I prayed to someday have two breasts again. I prayed for no more infections. I prayed that I would not go bankrupt. If it could be prayed for, I prayed for it.

CHAPTER 9

A God-Given Lifeline

Looking back over that 16-month journey, there was no question that my friends, colleagues, aunt, cousin, brother, and the doctors on my mini medical advisory board all provided tangible tools and insights to support this venture. My husband was also there every step of the way. From surgery and medical complications to legal advice and even packaging and shipping shirts, he was a steadfast supporter throughout. Together, they helped bring The Shower Shirt™ to market.

But beyond all of that, there was something else, something intangible. Something spiritual.

I consistently felt God's presence. Every step of the way, every decision, every obstacle, every small victory, I sensed guidance. I depended on blind faith throughout those 16 months. That's why I've always called The Shower Shirt™, *"A God product."* I was simply the liaison making it happen; God drove the vehicle.

At the time, and even now as I reflect on that period, I often ask myself what I truly learned from that journey. First and foremost, I learned how blessed I was to have friends, family, a husband, and colleagues who supported me, loved me, and refused to let me give up. I also realized how spiritually graced I was to feel the ongoing presence of my mother, whose guidance and love have never truly left me.

That understanding led to an even deeper realization: I had been in control the entire time because God was beside me, supporting me. I was just as much in control on that cold December day when my mother died as I was on the warm June day when I was diagnosed with breast cancer. I could not control the circumstances, but I could decide whether those experiences would break me or shape me, destroy me or strengthen me. In my mind, there was no choice. Giving up was easy. Growing, learning, and persevering were difficult. And it was never in my nature to surrender to anything or anyone. Fortunately, I found the source of strength, growth, and purpose to face my challenges.

I had always been a person of faith, but breast cancer and this project took me to a place of complete trust in blind faith. Creating The Shower Shirt™ became an act of surrender to something far greater than myself. I felt like an intermediary for a larger purpose, guided by forces beyond my understanding. Those deeply traumatic experiences, losing my mother, facing cancer, and enduring life-threatening infections, not only made me mentally and emotionally stronger, but also reaffirmed my faith and spirituality.

But before I reached that clarity, something extraordinary happened.

One evening, long before 500 units were sold, long before the patent was awarded, and long before I was healthy enough to work a full day, I lay in bed crying. I said out loud, *"I quit. I can't do this anymore. I am sick. I can't get rid of these infections. How can I create a product when I can't even work a full day?"*

Then, without warning, a strong, bass-like voice answered:
"Lisa, keep doing what you are doing."

I shouted back impulsively, *"I have no idea what I'm doing!"*

The voice repeated, calm but firm: *"Lisa, keep doing what you're doing."*

Frustrated, exhausted, and impatient, I responded again, *"I have no idea what I'm doing!"*

For a moment, I thought I was losing my mind. Then I wondered if I was simply exhausted, hallucinating from fatigue. But after a few minutes, I remembered my grandmother Crites, who often said that miracles happen every day, we just need to pay attention, to watch and listen for the signs.

I chose to accept the voice for what it was: a higher power. God was comforting me in my weakest moment. He was reminding me that He was present, that He understood my pain, and that I was not alone in trying to create something meaningful while still battling illness.

That day had been overwhelming. That night, I had said, *"I quit,"* and God heard me. He responded clearly, firmly, and unmistakably.

That evening changed everything.

Afterward, I stopped focusing on feeling sorry for myself and began focusing on transforming heartbreak into something meaningful. The Shower Shirt™ was never about me; it was about helping others.

I removed myself from the equation. This was about helping my friends and family, and ultimately, hundreds of thousands of breast cancer patients recover with dignity. It was about creating something that should have existed years earlier, but hadn't, because no one had taken it all the way through.

I began to see the product differently. It wasn't just a garment; it was a service, a way to support the women who would become my sisters. It was a way to transform months of pain into something purposeful. With that shift, the mission became mentally easier, the purpose clearer, and the faith that had carried me all along became something I could finally grasp.

The Shower Shirt™ became my God-given lifeline during those months of infections and hyperbaric treatments. It was more than a product; it felt like a child I had brought into the world. And in return, it gave me a reason to keep moving forward when everything else felt overwhelming. I was exhausted by doctors, hospitals, surgeries, and surgical drains. Every day carried frustration and fear. But The Shower Shirt™ became my therapy. It kept me from slipping into self-pity and gave me a sense of purpose and control that nothing else could.

Before that first voice told me to *"keep doing what you are doing,"* I had spent months on short-term disability, dealing with the emotional roller coaster of the unknown, barely able to eat, sleep, or sit through hyperbaric treatments. I missed my mother terribly. I was a furious forty-two-year-old, angry that she wasn't there to support me through this crisis. Angry that I was facing breast cancer so young. I missed my old life, my colleagues, and even felt guilty that coworkers had to cover my media work. I missed the gym, yoga, and biking to Port Canaveral, my Saturday morning ritual. In my early forties, I learned what it truly meant to value good health because once it was gone, its importance became undeniable.

A few months later, after another extremely difficult day with my recovery, while lying in bed upset, I heard another voice. This one was different, gentler, nurturing.

"Lisa, this is all going to be okay. I promise. You are worried and upset for no reason. This too shall pass."

I knew immediately it was my mother. She had said those exact words throughout my childhood. The voice was unmistakable, warm, loving, reassuring. Exactly what I needed to hear.

Over time, there were still days when fear, anxiety, and depression kept me in bed. But the voices persisted: *"Keep doing what you are doing. This too shall pass."*

Eventually, it didn't matter who was speaking. The fact that these moments continued was enough. I knew that if I abandoned this project, I would let my mother down and, most importantly, I would let God down.

Those voices gave me strength. They reminded me to focus on what I could gain and the opportunity to help others, rather than what I had lost. Over time, they helped me move forward with unwavering resolve.

In the years since, I have received countless messages, calls, emails, and texts from patients who have used The Shower

Shirt™. It's difficult to describe the joy I still feel when I read their testimonials. At times, it felt as though they were complimenting my child. I had nurtured this idea from concept to creation, and from creation to market. Every message felt personal.

Some came from physicians recommending the product. Others from dialysis patients using it for months at a time. Many were from breast cancer patients navigating surgery and reconstruction. Each message made me smile; some brought me to tears.

One message, in particular, was deeply emotional. A young woman wrote that her mother had passed away from a systemic infection caused by bacteria entering a post-surgical drain through bathwater. She said that if her mother had been able to use my invention, she might still be alive. I read her words and felt her grief in a way only someone who has lost a mother can understand. I cried for her and for myself.

Another person wrote simply, *"The Shower Shirt™ was a Godsend."* I responded, *"It's not just a Godsend. It's a God product. I believe He guided me every step of the way."*

We brought The Shower Shirt™ to market within 16 months of my breast cancer diagnosis and mastectomy. In research and development, that timeline is almost unheard of. I was not a trained researcher, developer, inventor, or entrepreneur. I was simply a breast cancer patient who believed in extraordinary timelines, driven by the conviction that future patients deserved the dignity I had fought so hard to reclaim.

CHAPTER 10

Who Knew a Shirt Could Do This?

Within a remarkably short time after going to market, The Shower Shirt™ had not only secured its benchmark patent for design and method of use, but had also obtained a trademarked logo and achieved Class 1 Medical Device classification. It was incredible to see something that began as a desperate idea, born out of my own need, recognized in every official capacity that mattered.

The SHOWER SHIRT

Over the years, extraordinary things continued to happen, expanding the reach and visibility of the product.

In 2015, I was honored to win an award at the National InnovateHER Challenge, sponsored by the U.S. Small Business Administration, The Washington Post, and Microsoft. The competition focused on women creating innovative products to support other women.

That recognition opened doors I had never imagined. Soon after, I was invited to present at WE-APEC, the Asia-

Pacific Economic Conference in Singapore, as a guest of the U.S. State Department.

That same year, I received the Patient Innovation Award from the University of Portugal and the Católica School of Business and Economics. I was among the first award recipients, at a time when the program was still in its early stages. Founded by Pedro Oliveira, PhD, and Helena Canhao, MD, the initiative has since expanded significantly, both nationally and internationally. The program now includes professors from institutions across the globe, including Harvard, MIT, New York University, and Berkeley, all serving on its board of directors.

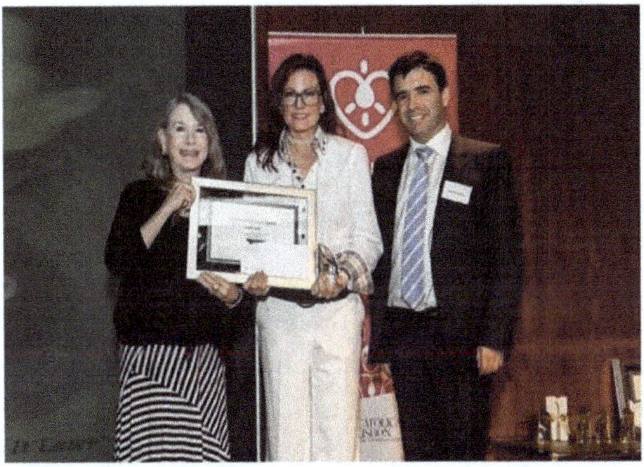

From left to right: Dr. Carliss Baldwin from Harvard University, me, and Dr. Pedro Olivera at the Patient Innovation Awards ceremony – Lisbon, Portugal

At the Lisbon award ceremony, MIT professor Dr. Eric von Hippel helped me understand why The Shower Shirt™ had never existed before I created it. During his presentation, titled *"Why Innovation Doesn't Always Come from Industry,"* he asked the audience, *"Why is it that Lisa Crites invented The Shower Shirt™, while the medical industry did not, even after years of clear need?"*

The answer was simple. The medical industry focused on numbers and the bottom line. I did not. I created innovation based on emotion and patient need, not profit. That insight inspired me to write a column in *Florida Today* titled *"Not All Progress Comes from Industry,"* quoting Dr. von Hippel. It was, in part, a critique of the profit-driven nature of healthcare, but it was also an honest reflection of my experience.

Because of that recognition in Portugal, The Shower Shirt™ is now on display in the London Science Museum's Science Innovation Exhibit, which spans seventy-eight locations across Europe. As the award was academic in nature, it also led to interviews for several academic doctoral theses and published books focused on patient-driven innovation.

The accolades continued. I was later invited to present The Shower Shirt™ at the World Government Summit in Dubai, at the Edge of Government exhibit, as a guest of Sheikh Mohammad. During that trip, I interviewed Shatha Alhashmi, a professor and employee from the Prime Minister's office, who shared insights into the expanding opportunities for women in business in Dubai. With her perspective, I wrote another column for the Florida Today and USA Network titled *"Business and the Burqa,"* reflecting on my experience at the summit.

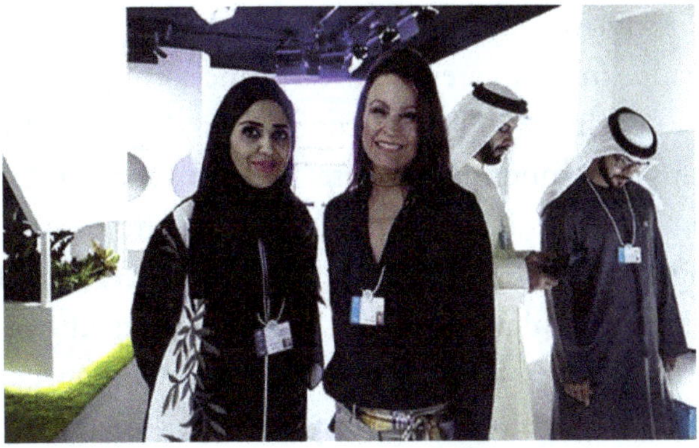

Shatha Alhashmi and Me at the World Government Summit

During the Dubai trip, we appeared on Dubai TV. I could not understand the language, but a bilingual friend assured me the coverage was very positive. Soon after, Amazon corporate reached out with interest in hosting the product online. Hospital gift shops, mastectomy boutiques, and breast cancer support groups continued to follow, all eager to offer The Shower Shirt™ directly to patients.

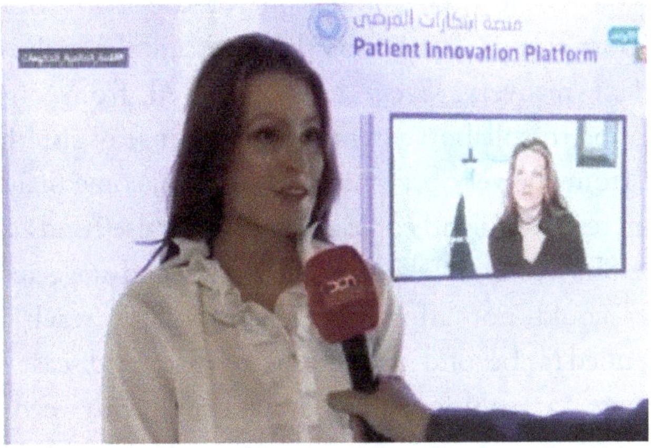

Featured on Dubai TV

Driven by Heart in Florida and the Zonta Club of Defiance in Ohio are two breast cancer support organizations with which we collaborated for more than a decade. Both groups raise funds to purchase The Shower Shirt™ and donate it to patients and local hospital systems. The Zonta Club works alongside OKuley's Pharmacy, Mercy Health, and ProMedica Regional Hospital to identify women undergoing breast cancer treatment. Their efforts are consistent, providing Tools Needed Through Transformation (TNT) bags to patients across the United States.

I have deep admiration for the many breast cancer support groups nationwide that dedicate themselves to easing patient recovery. Every call I received from organizations wanting to collaborate reinforced the sense of sisterhood I had felt from the very beginning. Over time, some dialysis centers also created philanthropic programs to raise funds and donate The Shower Shirt™ to patients with end-stage renal disease who could not afford it. The product's reach eventually extended far beyond mastectomy and kidney disease patients. It became a solution for individuals with central lines, chemotherapy pumps, wound vacs, external defibrillators, and those recovering from chest or abdominal surgeries, including cardiac patients undergoing pacemaker battery replacement. Over fourteen years, The Shower Shirt™ has been shipped to Canada, England, Ireland, Spain, Australia, New Zealand, Austria, Japan, Israel, Brazil, the Seychelles, Dubai, and every state in the United States.

Since the beginning of this journey, opportunities have continued to follow because of The Shower Shirt™. The people I have met and the places I have traveled have been life changing. In 2024, I was nominated for induction into the Florida Inventors Hall of Fame. In 2025, I presented on the Necessity Driven Innovators Panel for the United States Patent and Trademark Office.

That same year, after more than a decade, I finally met my manufacturing partners in person. I traveled to Asia and met Lynn from MEELYNN Garment Company. There were no Zoom calls or WhatsApp messages. We were in the same place at the same time. I was thrilled to meet the person who had worked tirelessly, year after year, to manufacture The Shower Shirt™. While in Hong Kong, she shared something that deeply moved me. She had always believed in my mission to help breast cancer patients, and that belief was the reason she remained flexible over the years, accommodating smaller production runs that did not always make business sense.

As we spent the day together, I kept thinking about how our connection had begun more than ten years earlier, long before we had ever met in person. When you remove borders and set aside governments, the tensions between countries fade. What remains is simple. Two women from different parts of the world, working toward the same purpose, which was to make life easier for other women.

I felt immense gratitude, not only for finally meeting her, but for the opportunity to thank her face to face for believing in my mission from the very beginning.

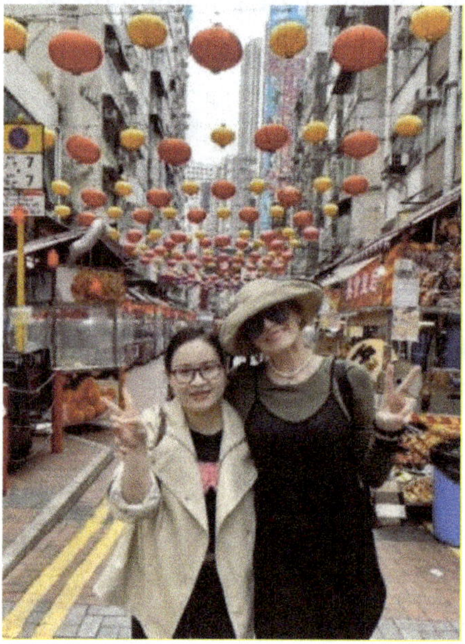

Me and Lynn in Hong Kong.

CHAPTER 11

Penile Implants Necessary – Breast Cancer Debated?

The Essentially Women conference had been exhilarating. But amid the media attention, product demonstrations, and networking, one issue loomed over me like a cloud: securing a dedicated HCPCS code for The Shower Shirt™. Without it, no one, whether a breast cancer patient or a dialysis patient, could have the shirt covered by Medicare, Medicaid, or commercial insurers.

I had no idea how vast and complex this process would be. We were starting at ground zero. No product like mine had ever existed, especially from a regulatory standpoint. In the world of insurance reimbursement, Medicare was the gatekeeper. If Medicare did not approve it, commercial insurers would not even consider it.

So I applied for an individual HCPCS code through the Centers for Medicare and Medicaid Services. The first response came back quickly. Denied. The reason was that existing Medicare policy stated breast cancer and mastectomy patients were not eligible for reimbursement for shower coverings because they were not considered medically necessary.

Not medically necessary?

Under Medicare guidelines, a service or product is medically necessary if it protects or improves a patient's health and if its absence could negatively affect the patient's condition, based on accepted medical standards.

That made no sense to me. The Shower Shirt™ was specifically designed to protect a patient's health and prevent complications. Without it, the risk to the patient could absolutely increase.

I did not give up. I revised my application, expanding it to include additional patient populations using The Shower Shirt™. Dialysis patients, cardiac patients, and those recovering from chest and abdominal surgeries. Then I applied again.

Another denial.

This time, however, the committee offered me something I had only imagined. I was invited to present before the CMS HCPCS Committee on Capitol Hill and advocate for coverage. My stomach dropped. Lobbying in Washington, D.C.? Me? I had no idea what I was doing.

Fortunately, my attorney's firm, helping with the HCPCS process resided in Washington and thrilled by the request to present. They accompanied me and arranged transportation to the CMS building. But first came security. Cars were stopped and scanned for explosives. Guards checked underneath vehicles with flashlights. We were told certain cars could not park anywhere near the building. At one point, we were miles from the entrance, standing in the summer heat. After hours of screening, walking, and waiting, we were finally dropped at the front door.

I remember thinking, take a deep breath. Maybe this will be quick. Maybe I will be one of the first to present.

I was not. I was twentieth out of twenty-five.

One by one, CEOs and presidents from large, well-known healthcare and medical device companies made their cases. Each argued why their product deserved a HCPCS code. Time dragged on. I tried to calm myself. I did yoga in the bathroom, meditated, even jogged in place. Nothing worked. Eventually, I went outside, sat on the steps, and prayed.

God, calm me. Help me get through this. Let me speak clearly.

A sense of calm slowly settled over me, and I realized that I could do this. I walked back inside, focused, and approached the podium.

My intuition told me to direct my attention to the men on the panel, many of whom avoided eye contact. There were eight women and five men. The women looked engaged, some even nodding. The men looked uncomfortable.

I leaned forward slightly, met their eyes, and asked the question that had been circling in my mind for months:

"Would you want your mother, sister, or daughter standing in the shower with a trash bag after breast cancer and amputation of the breasts? Or would you rather they use a product designed to protect surgical drain sites after mastectomy surgery?"

The reaction was immediate. The men shifted in their seats, glanced at one another, flushed, and quickly looked away.

In that moment, I realized many of them had no understanding of the clinical reality of mastectomy recovery. Trash bags. Tape. Plastic wrap. Women trying to shower while managing surgical drains. Yet they were responsible for deciding which medical products deserved reimbursement.

As I continued, I stayed grounded in my talking points. I cited infection data from the American Hospital Association and explained how waterborne infections after surgery could significantly increase costs for Medicare and insurers. Then I shared my story.

I am a breast cancer survivor, I told them. Every patient deserves better than a trash bag after amputation of the breasts. That is why I created this product.

I went on to describe the patient populations using The Shower Shirt™, the infections it was designed to help prevent, the dignity it restored, and the reality that many patients had no alternative. I was not pleading. I was presenting facts with clarity, urgency, and just enough emotion to help them picture someone they loved in that position.

By the time I finished, I was not sure whether they were convinced or simply uncomfortable. But I had said what needed to be said. I had shown up, in a suit and heels, with my nerves shaking, and told the panel exactly what was at stake: human dignity, patient safety, and a product born from necessity, not profit.

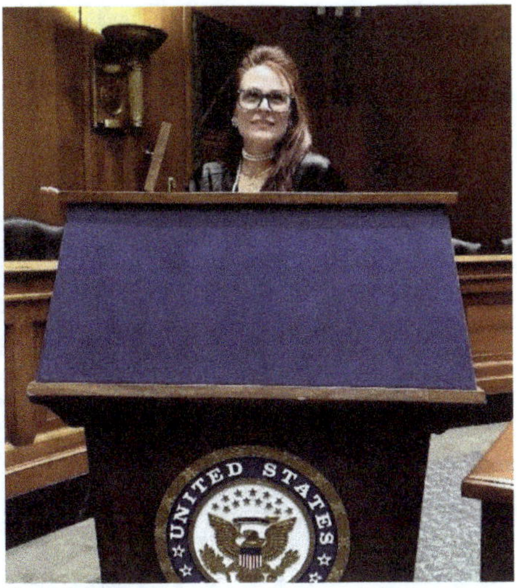

Me Speaking at CMS

The women on the committee gave me brief smiles when I asked my pointed questions. They immediately understood who I was fighting for, and why. Not just for breast cancer patients, but for every woman on that panel and every woman in the country. Their nods and quiet *"atta girl"* expressions made me feel like I had an army behind me, even if it was only the women in that room.

Meanwhile, the men continued to fidget and avoided eye contact. In another setting, it might have been funny, but in that moment, it was frustrating. Later that week, I appeared on WUSA, the CBS affiliate in Washington, D.C., to express my disappointment that after two denials, Medicare still would not cover any protective showering product for breast cancer patients. I had learned that even something as basic as a post-mastectomy shower garment would require an act of Congress to gain coverage.

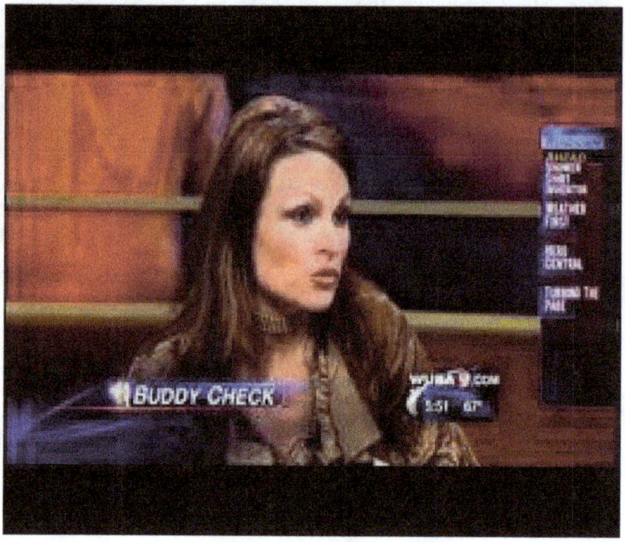

CBS in Washington DC

While I was in Washington preparing that presentation with my attorneys, I came across something that made me stop and stare. As I reviewed the policy details, I discovered that penile implants are covered under Medicare. In other words, they are officially considered medically necessary for men.

I went back and read the line again to make sure I had not misunderstood it. I remember thinking, wait, seriously? I did not know whether to laugh at the irony or feel frustrated by what it implied.

The government was willing to pay significant amounts for devices for male genitalia, yet would not reimburse a protective garment that could help reduce the risk of waterborne infections in post-surgical patients, which would ultimately save money. I did not let that contradiction go unaddressed. I raised it directly with the committee and later during the CBS interview. It also explained why the men had avoided eye contact during my questions.

Soon after my presentation, a woman named J. Lundquist reached out to me. She became an invaluable resource, researching the *"protective showering"* category. She discovered that Medicare already covered showering garments for the end-stage renal disease population, those undergoing dialysis, under a bundled reimbursement rate. This provided at least a foundation, a set of talking points, and a possible pathway toward broader reimbursement.

I immediately contacted Congressman Bill Posey, our district representative, and asked for his help. His congressional liaisons began working with J. Lundquist's office to better understand the issue. Both Congressman Posey and Senator Bill Nelson wrote letters supporting the need for Medicare coverage for a protective product for breast cancer patients. But support and action are two vastly different things.

One day, Ms. Lundquist called and said, *"Your congressional liaisons keep contacting us about this application. If they want shower coverings for breast cancer patients to be reimbursed, they need to file legislation."* She explained it clearly. There was no alternative path. Legislative action was the only option.

With the help of my friend Dr. Stephanie Haridopolos, whose husband Mike had served for years in the Florida Senate, we arranged a meeting with Congressman Posey's office. That meeting led to additional trips to Washington, including discussions with Vice President Joe Biden's Chief of Staff and teams from both Congressman Posey's office and

Congresswoman Debbie Wasserman Schultz's office. Eventually, legislation was introduced: the Post-Mastectomy Infection Reduction Act, created to secure Medicare coverage for shower garments for breast cancer patients.

On Friday, May 9, 2014, bipartisan legislation was introduced by U.S. Representatives Bill Posey and Debbie Wasserman Schultz to support breast cancer patients during recovery after surgery. The Post-Mastectomy Infection Reduction Act, H.R. 4627, authorized Medicare to extend coverage for these garments when deemed medically necessary to reduce the risk of infection.

Months of navigating bureaucracy finally led to political support. And the lesson I took from it was simple. Never give up. Keep pushing, keep speaking, and yes, be the squeaky wheel, but manage the tone. As my friend Stephon Williams, a life coach, often says, remember to PUSH, Push Until Something Happens. That is exactly what I did.

To celebrate this milestone, I attended an Inventors Conference on Capitol Hill. It provided an opportunity to discuss the legislation with congressional staff, Senate leaders, and the media.

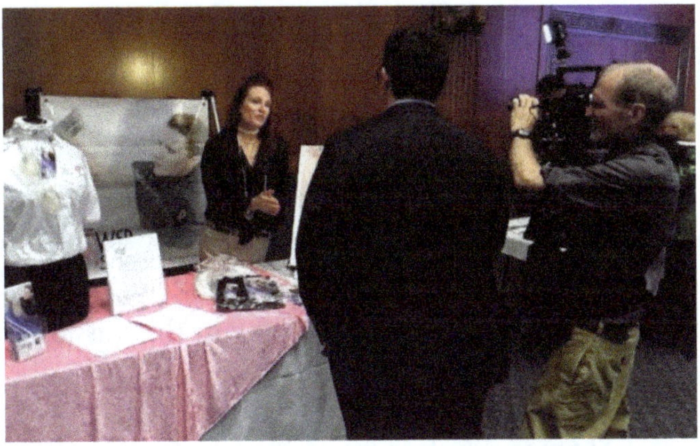

Capitol Hill Inventors Conference

To keep the media engaged in the filing of legislation, I wrote yet another print column for *Florida Today* and USA Network titled "Medicare Reimbursement Battle Progresses," explaining that sometimes it literally takes an act of Congress to keep women out of trash bags after mastectomy surgery.

With legislation filed, I refocused on the business. Since The Shower Shirt™ was already covered for dialysis patients under the ESRD composite payment bundle, under HCPCS code A9270, we began marketing to the National Kidney Foundation and attending related conferences. Dialysis patients soon began reaching out.

I remember one call vividly. A woman in Rockledge, Florida, who lived close by, needed a Shower Shirt for her daughter, who was acutely diabetic and undergoing dialysis. Because she lived nearby, I decided to deliver the order in person. Mrs. King was kind and warm, but clearly exhausted and emotional, balancing her love for her daughter with the reality of her chronic illness. She showed me how she planned to modify the shirt to fit her daughter, who was a 3X plus size, since the largest size we offered would have been snug.

I will never forget that visit. Her dedication, care, and love were tangible. Afterward, she stayed in touch, sending photos of her daughter wearing the newly adapted, cape-like Shower Shirt. It was moments like that, seeing the product help someone directly, that reminded me why this mission was bigger than me.

Six months after my visit with the Kings, I received a note. My heart sank as I read the words. Her daughter had passed away *"at the tender age of 39."* But then she wrote something that has stayed with me ever since: *"Thank you for your contribution in helping my daughter shower the last few months of her life."*

That note hit me harder than I expected. At the same time, it reminded me exactly why I had been pushing The Shower Shirt™ forward, battling bureaucracy, HCPCS committees, infections, and fatigue. That was why I kept going, for the moments that mattered most to real people, for the lives we could touch, even in small but meaningful ways. It was also because of Mrs. King's daughter that we soon expanded plus sizing for the product, so no caregiver would need to modify the garment again.

I had also finally neared the end of my reconstruction journey. Dr. Z returned to replace the right breast with a final implant, and thankfully, everything went smoothly. Six months later, the left tissue expander was replaced with the final implant. Because of my history with infections on that side, I returned to hyperbaric treatments for a month, along with prophylactic antibiotics, just to be safe. Finally, I had two breasts again.

Yes, I could finally look in the mirror and see two, albeit heavily scarred, breasts. But there were limits. My surgeon could not complete the tattooing process to recreate the appearance of nipples. The risk was simply too high. The left breast had already been problematic, and the team was concerned that even minor tattooing could trigger another infection. So we stopped there, choosing caution over completion.

It felt surreal to be whole again, and most importantly, my schedule began to normalize. My immune system was finally strong enough to go out without constant worry. I could visit friends, socialize, bike, and finally get back in the gym. But jogging was out of the question. I still had what I call False Emotions Appearing Real, or FEAR. Seeing more than 300,000 women undergo breast augmentation each year, I know implants are generally safe. But reactive implants after breast cancer and infections are a different reality, and I remained focused on protecting what I had fought so hard to regain.

Even now, years later, I cannot shake the thought of jogging with implants. I imagine MRSA returning and sending me back into the hyperbaric chamber. I protect my implants like precious cargo because, to me, they are. They represent survival, resilience, and every patient I have tried to help along the way.

Not long ago, I came across an old song by Kenny Loggins titled *"Conviction of the Heart."* The song had been around since my college days in the 1980s, when Footloose was the soundtrack of life. Back then, I hardly paid attention to its meaning. But watching the video years later, the message struck me differently. It spoke about conviction and about doing something meaningful from the deepest place in your heart.

Listening to it again, I realized this has been my journey since 2009. I have carried a conviction of the heart to protect women recovering from breast cancer surgery, to ensure no one has to go through what I experienced. I had a conviction to create something that allows patients to heal with dignity. One line from the song resonates deeply: *"The growth of consciousness does not depend on the might of the intellect, but on conviction of the heart."* There is nothing more powerful than the determination to pursue what your heart genuinely believes in.

Helping people is the greatest victory there is. No amount of money or recognition compares to the fulfillment of easing someone's pain or helping them feel whole again. That is what true success feels like.

Over the years, I have carried this belief into every part of my life. I have served on nonprofit boards, including the Historic Cocoa Village Playhouse, Digital Arts for Autism, Driven by Heart, and Space Coast Early Steps. I have volunteered with the Second Harvest Food Bank of Central Florida and the Central Florida Homeless Coalition. Most recently, I joined the advisory board for weVenture, the Women's Business Center at the Florida Institute of Technology. Each of these experiences has deepened my understanding of what it means to live with purpose.

Sir Winston Churchill once said, "*We make a living by what we earn, but we make a life by what we give.*" I have found those words to be one of the truest measures of success. Giving refines us. In the end, it defines the legacy we leave behind.

I always said I never wanted breast cancer to 'define' my life, but hoped it somehow could 'refine' my life. In looking back, somewhere between the ups and downs, tears, disappointments and triumphs, I believe it has.

CHAPTER 12

Driven By Heart

By now, The Shower Shirt™ had been on the market for a couple of years and had started to make a name for itself in our local community. Finally, we were seeing a small, exceedingly small, profit. But I quickly learned that running a business was expensive. Between ongoing FDA and patent licensing costs, the legal costs in fighting for Medicare coverage, product liability insurance, manufacturing, shipping, tariffs, and the usual overhead that comes with any business, there was not much left at the end of the day.

Still, I felt the company could finally give back and support something related to breast cancer. After everything I had endured clinically, I knew I needed to pay it forward in some way, though I was not yet sure how. I could not donate a large sum of money, but maybe I could help in a small, tangible way, such as donating shirts to patients who could not afford one.

That is when a new group of sisters entered my life.

I reached out to a local breast cancer support group called Breast Friends of Florida, part of the national Breast Friends organization based in Oregon, hoping to explore a collaboration. From the start, I connected immediately with the executive directors, Sherry Palmer and Connie Chiles-Cooke. We shared something profound. We were all breast cancer survivors. It did not take long for me to learn that the entire board of directors were survivors as well, which was a requirement for serving. I realized this was another kind of sisterhood, one dedicated to supporting hundreds of local breast cancer patients from diagnosis through recovery.

Sherry and Connie shared their stories with me. When they had gone through breast cancer just a few years earlier, they had done it mostly alone. Surgeons, nurses, and occasionally social workers were there for the clinical side, but no one was there to guide them through the emotional experience or help them understand what would come next. No one explained the small but critical details of recovery or the practical realities and side effects of treatment. Sherry put it simply: *"There was not one person to say, 'Yes, it is absolutely normal to feel this way."*

She added, *"No one told me I should avoid the dentist or skip a manicure or pedicure because of infection risk during treatment. Some tips may appear in pamphlets, but having someone explain how to navigate life during surgery, radiation, and chemotherapy is priceless."*

I understood completely. I had faced the same isolation. No one had prepared me for the infections, the confusion, the emotional trauma, or the panic that came with it. With Dr. Z limiting time with me due to ongoing complications, I often felt completely alone, just as Sherry and Connie had.

Soon after that meeting, I was invited to join the board of directors. From the very first meetings, I saw firsthand the difference this team was making in the lives of breast cancer patients. It was one thing to hear about their work. It was another to witness it up close. The comfort they provided, the guidance they offered, and the hope they instilled were undeniable. I knew immediately that this chapter of *Beautifully Unbroken* needed to reflect their journey.

Over time, Breast Friends of Florida evolved into a new organization, Driven By Heart, led by Sherry Palmer. With the unifying theme "Fighting Breast Cancer Together," the group expanded beyond the local community. They grew through corporate partnerships and strengthened their network by bringing surgeons, oncologists, and general practitioners onto their advisory board. Before long, women from across the country were reaching out for support. In response, the team began mailing care packages to breast cancer patients nationwide.

These were not ordinary packages. Along with thoughtful support items, they created personalized bags for each patient. Every bag included practical tools to ease surgery and help manage the exhausting side effects of chemotherapy, from soft blankets to post-surgical essentials. Their goal was simple but powerful: to make the journey a little more manageable and a little less lonely. I related to this deeply because it aligned with the mission behind The Shower Shirt™, helping women regain comfort, dignity, and a sense of normalcy during an overwhelming medical experience.

Since 2009, the organization has become a trusted referral resource for the clinical community, including doctors, nurses, breast navigators, and surgeons. To date, the 501(c)(3) nonprofit has supported more than 4,500 women in our community, with that number continuing to grow each month. Driven By Heart has been sustained for more than sixteen years through fundraising, donations, and a dedicated network of volunteers. Every support group session, every post-surgical bra, every drain holder, and every Shower Shirt is provided to patients free of charge.

The story of Driven By Heart mirrors the story behind The Shower Shirt™. At its core, both are about people helping people, women supporting women, and breast cancer patients lifting each other up. Every journey through breast cancer is different, and the unknown can be overwhelming. Some patients face it with little support from family or friends. Others struggle simply because they lack access to the right information or guidance. That is where this remarkable group steps in. They are advocates, caregivers, and sisters in the truest sense.

This is a club none of us ever wanted to join. Yet once we are in it, we find understanding, support, and connection from others who have walked the same path. Because of Driven By Heart, women facing breast cancer in Brevard County, Florida, have a place to turn. A safe and compassionate space where they are guided, supported, and reminded that they are not alone.

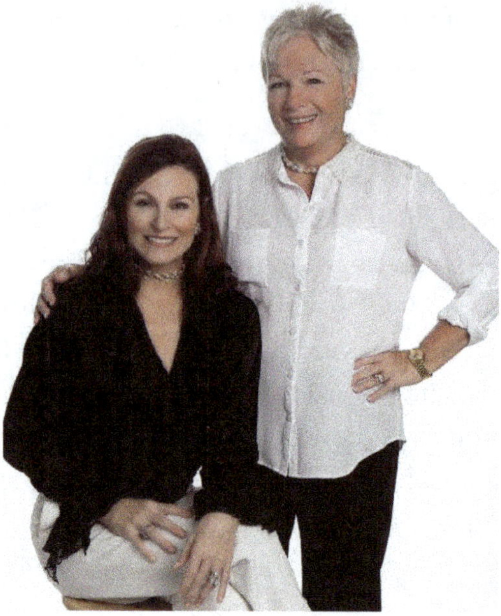

Me and Sherry Palmer, Driven By Heart, Executive Director, from a Space Coast Living Magazine feature

CHAPTER 13

God's Hands Around Me

As my grandmother Crites would say, *"There are miracles which happen daily, we just need to pay attention, watch, and listen for those miraculous moments."* I have carried her words with me throughout my life, believing that when we ask, God places His hands on us and wraps His arms around us every day. We need only be open-minded enough to feel His touch, attentive enough to see His actions, and aware enough to hear His voice.

As you may already know, since I have mentioned it a time or two, I am a true Midwest farm girl. I grew up in the Methodist Church in a small town, right in what some folks call the Bible Belt. That is a nickname for areas with strong evangelical Protestant traditions, conservative values, and a deep emphasis on faith. Life there revolved around school, church, family, and friends. It felt like a real-life Mayberry, full of large farming families and good Christian people. On Sunday mornings, the faces at church were the same ones I saw at school, from teachers to parents to friends, all woven together in a close-knit community.

Over the years, I found myself evolving into more of a spiritual person than a religious one. I came to see spirituality as an internal journey, focused on personal and subjective paths to meaning, purpose, and connection to something greater. As I matured, spirituality became my creative force. Organized religion had guided me toward structured beliefs, rituals, and shared practices, but spirituality offered me freedom. I still value the purpose of organized religion, yet I have learned that, like healthcare, it can sometimes function more as a business than a ministry. I have observed some religious organizations where structure and financial priorities overshadow the human experience. As a free thinker, I found the institutional focus of religion limiting for my spirit.

My parents were not fond of me sharing that personal evolution, so I kept it mostly to myself. At an early age, I learned that being outspoken about politics or any contrasting viewpoints related to religion did not go over well in the Crites household. Still, spirituality remained my anchor. It has kept me grounded in gratitude, supported my creativity, and nurtured a deep appreciation for every blessing in my life.

I had always believed in miracles. But it was only at the funeral home after my mother's death that I truly understood what it meant for God to have His hands on me and His arms wrapped around me.

I had been married for only two weeks and had just returned from our honeymoon when we learned of my mother's fatal accident. My husband and I immediately flew back to the Midwest. I remember wanting to speak with Reverend Vaughn Wright, the preacher who had just married us at the First Christian Church. He was tall, calm, and composed, with a presence that conveyed both strength and peace. I felt an urgent need to meet with him. I needed him to tell me that my mother still cared about what was happening here on earth after she had passed. For some reason, I felt she had abandoned us. In my mind, when someone leaves, they no longer care. I knew it was irrational, but grief can make the irrational feel real.

When I met with Reverend Wright, he was kind and patient. However, he did not say what I needed to hear. Instead, he spoke about theology and the teachings of heaven, repeating that *"there will be no sorrow in heaven."* I left his office convinced that my mother no longer cared. She had moved on to everlasting life, and I was left to carry the grief of my father, my three brothers, and myself.

I went to the funeral home and spoke with Greg Mathis, the owner, who had known my family all my life. I told him I needed time with my mother over the next few days and that I wanted to do her makeup. I had always done her makeup for important occasions, including my own wedding just two weeks earlier, so it felt right to do it one last time. After some discussion, Greg agreed.

For two long days, I sat beside my mother. I finished her makeup, told her she had been the best mother, and expressed how grateful I was to be her daughter. Most importantly, I spoke to her about my need to know she was okay and that she still cared for us, even though she was no longer physically present. I asked for a sign. I sat beside her casket for hours, sometimes into the evening, while my cousin Mandy and my husband waited in the next room. My father called repeatedly, asking me to come home, but I kept saying, *"No, I want to be with Mom."*

On the morning of the funeral, I arrived early, just as the day was beginning. My friend Barbara, my best friend since third grade, was with me. She was already there, standing in the quiet before anyone else arrived. She moved around the room, taking pictures of the hundreds of bouquets and floral arrangements. I sat beside my mother and spoke softly to her, telling her that visitation would begin soon, followed by the funeral and then the cemetery, where she would be laid to rest near her parents and grandparents. I reminded her that my physical time with her was almost gone.

Suddenly, I felt an urge to place my hand on the left side of her chest. The moment I did, I felt warmth. It caught me off guard. It was a cold December morning, two days before Christmas, and the room was cool. Why did her chest feel warm?

I moved my hand across her chest, near her collarbone, which I knew had been broken in the accident. Each time my hand passed over the area where the heart rests, I felt that same warmth. It felt like the heat of a fever. I became completely focused on it. For nearly thirty minutes, I sat there with my hand on her chest, feeling that warmth. I checked other parts of her body, and they were cold. But that one area remained warm.

After a while, my husband David came over and said, *"Lisa, the family will be here soon. You need to wrap it up."* I asked him to feel her chest. He did, and in his usual calm, clinical tone said, *"Lisa, you asked for a sign, and you have one. The heart is closer to the center of the body, and blood is pumped from the left ventricle. You wanted a sign, and you got it. You need to wrap it up."*

His response was direct and unemotional, exactly as I expected. David is a serious, thoughtful Catholic, and his communication is always concise and grounded. He works in orthopedic medicine, and his clinical approach comes naturally to him.

Shortly after, my father and older brother Shawn arrived. I asked them to feel her chest as well, telling them I would explain later. They both confirmed the warmth.

That day, more than 1,500 people attended my mother's funeral in Dexter, Missouri, where she was raised. The turnout was not surprising. Her father had owned the local dairy. After marrying my father, she settled on the family farm nearby. She had been deeply involved in the community, serving on the Children's Home Board, the Economic Development Board, and as a regional representative for the Girl Scouts. She had touched many lives, which was reflected in the number of people who came to honor her.

At the time, I questioned everything I was experiencing. I looked to my husband, my father, and my brother for validation, wanting confirmation that what I felt was real. I even asked Mr. Mathis if there was any explanation for the warmth. He shook his head and said, "*No, Lisa. Your mom has been in a cooler for three days.*"

The experience was overwhelming at the moment. Only later did I fully understand its significance. The warmth I felt was a sign that my mother was okay. It was a message that she still cared about me, my brothers, and our lives, even though she was no longer physically present. It reaffirmed what my grandmother had always said: miracles happen every day, but we must be open to recognizing them.

That day at the funeral home was both simple and profound. God had given me the sign I needed, confirming that my mother was at peace. It reassured me that our beliefs about life after death were real. My mother was alive in spirit, and through that moment, I felt her presence and her love on the day we laid her to rest.

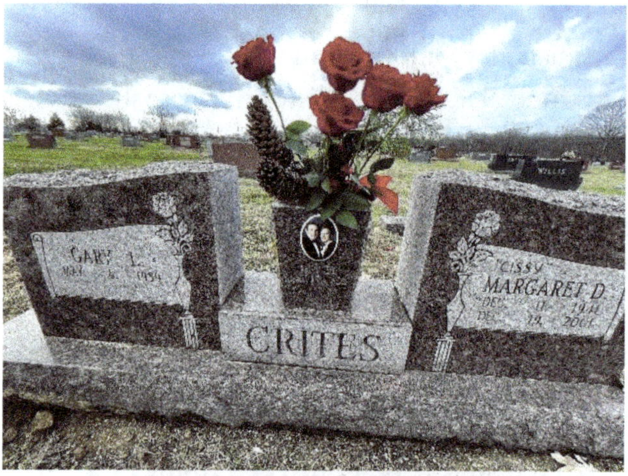

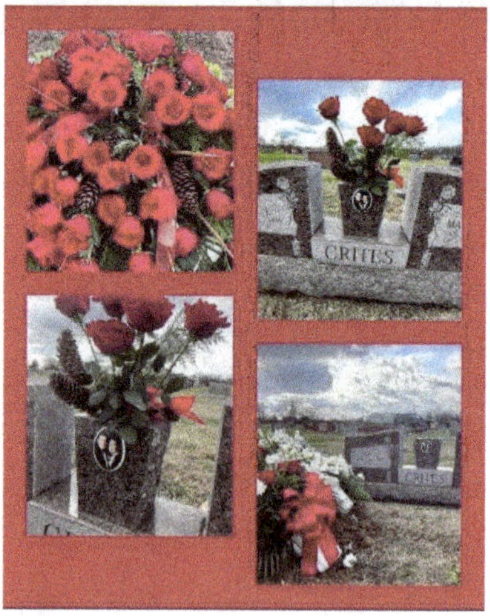

CHAPTER 14

When My Mother Spoke Again

Have you ever had a project you kept putting off? I had one that took me twenty-four years to finally tackle. Recently, while cleaning out a storage unit, I came across bins filled with my mother's keepsakes from junior high through high school. Back then, scrapbooks with cardboard pages were the perfect way to preserve dried flowers, ribbons, newspaper clippings, love notes, and, of course, photos and awards. My mother, who rarely threw anything away, had amassed a remarkable collection of these mementos, each one offering a small window into her early life.

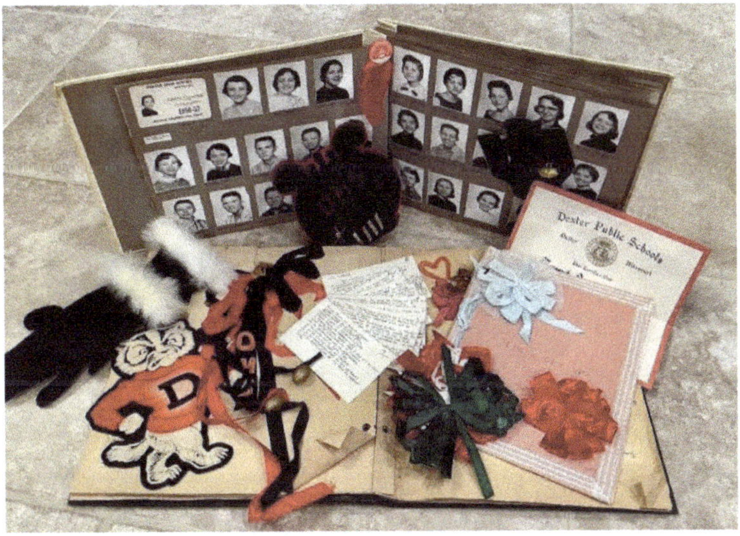

My mother's scrapbook belongings from the 1950's

My mother graduated from high school in 1959 and, as you know, was tragically killed in a car accident in 2001, a loss that had long fueled my procrastination and made this project feel even more daunting. When I saw the aged boxes, I immediately recognized what they were, and my heart sank. Yet after more than two decades, I found the strength to finally take it on.

Among the letters, photos, and yearbooks, I discovered an envelope labeled *"Cissy's Speech"* in my grandmother's handwriting, Cissy being my mother's nickname. A little investigation revealed that she had been appointed to an advisory role in a national girls' organization called The International Order of the Rainbow Girls, a Masonic youth service sorority dedicated to teaching leadership, character development, and community service to girls between the ages of 11 and 20.

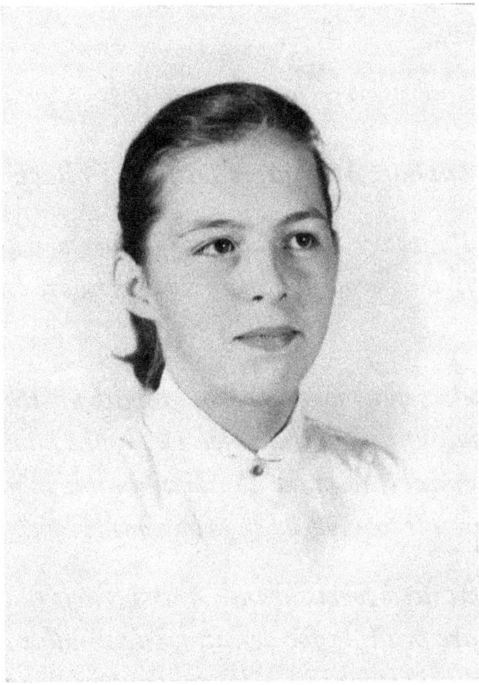

My mother at 18

The speech my mother gave at her induction ceremony, at the age of 18, was typed on a manual typewriter using 3 by 5 index cards. Reading it brought me to tears, and even my husband, who never met her, was moved. As I went through her words, I realized they were meant not only for her sorority sisters, but for young girls everywhere. That message feels just as important today, perhaps even more so than it did in 1959. Some of her phrases made me smile, like *"fellas"* and *"old man anxiety,"* a charming reminder of her time. What surprised me most was the depth of her Christian based reflections at such a youthful age. I knew it was important to include her words in this book as both inspiration and a glimpse into the young woman she was.

OUR VICTORY

Author: Margaret Dianne Pollock

God supplies the power that makes a Victory a reality, and as Rainbow Girls, tomorrow's wives and mothers, are ever searching for Victory.

We find ourselves quiet when we should speak up, timid when we should be brave, and doubtful when we should have faith. We find ourselves unable to make decisions, unable to stand for our beliefs, even unable to know when to love or not love.

We feel a great need for assurance, and without that assurance, often feel we are heading for defeat, while stumbling under the doubts and fears that we face. We are tempted to act upon what we know is evil and are often overcome with sorrow and disappointment afterward. We let envy and selfishness find a place in our life.

We face frustrations, anxieties, and worries. Everywhere we go, in everything we do, we come face-to-face with Old Man Anxiety. If only it will happen; if only the test is not hard, if only that fella would call. But if it does not happen, we are then left to a state of further anxiety, for then we let ourselves worry over the wrong that we have done and ignore our conscience.

We lack faith, belief, and trust to try, seek, and dare. We search for a victory that does not come.

Yet we can be victorious. We can stand with our heads high and our hearts proud, and we can overcome the many temptations we face. We can live happily and make those around us happy, too... We can live victoriously.

When doubt begins to creep into our minds and that doubt leads to another and another and our hearts become hard and our thoughts cynical, we need to remember that the way to victory is relatively simple: Believe in God, in his Son, in others, and ourselves and in great causes; and then, stand for those convictions and beliefs. Turn unbelief to belief, doubt to faith, questioning to questing, and from defeat to Victory – a positive Victory.

We must think happy thoughts, do happy things, and associate with happy people. There is no Victory in complaining and feeling sorry for oneself for the last battle is within oneself– and it is not an easy battle. But, if we have faith, if we have hope, if we have charity – in ourselves as well as in others' – there can be a victory.

Let us strive to live up to the ideals of the inspiring prayer of St. Frances of Assisi:

Where there is hatred—let us sow love.
Where there is injury – pardon.
Where there is doubt – faith.
Where there is despair – hope.
Where there is darkness – light.
Where there is sadness – joy.
O Divine Master, grant that I may not so much seek to be consoled – as to console.
To be understood – as to understand.
To be loved – as to love, for, it is in giving that we receive.

It is in pardoning – that we are pardoned.
It is in dying – that we are born to eternal life.

Of course, I am biased, but reading my mother's message from her teenage years brought smiles, laughter, and a stream of tears. At such a young age, she demonstrated a level of spiritual insight and wisdom that I did not acquire until much later, long after she had passed. I will always treasure this speech, all fifteen index cards, still in perfect condition, typed on a manual typewriter nearly seventy years ago. As they say in the world of antiques, *"What a find."*

CHAPTER 15

How I Accidentally Became a Keynote Speaker

Over the past few years, after gaining incredible print and television media coverage, along with accolades and awards highlighting me, The Shower Shirt™, and our mission, something unexpected started happening. I began receiving calls asking me to speak at breast cancer luncheons, fundraising events, and more. I was genuinely surprised. My first official invitation came from the Zonta Club of Defiance in Defiance, Ohio, for their annual fundraiser, and my initial reaction was, why would anyone want to pay me to speak?

The invitation came from a kind woman named Annette Kuhlman. Her mother had gone through breast cancer, and Annette had been her caregiver every step of the way. She understood the fear, the exhaustion, and the heartache. She had lived it. From our first conversation, I felt an immediate connection. Her mother had passed away at 61, and just like that, Annette became another sister in this unspoken club of women affected by this disease. On top of that, we shared the bond of being motherless daughters, which made it even more personal.

Still, I hesitated. Sharing my story with a live audience felt terrifying. I reached out to a friend from the National Speakers Bureau, and she, along with several friends and family members, encouraged me to move forward. They reminded me that my story mattered. But one question kept circling in my mind: why was I so afraid to tell it?

Every morning felt like a negotiation. Step one was getting out of bed. Step two was starting to write the script. And every day, I found a way to delay it. I was paralyzed. FEAR, False Emotions Appearing Real, had its grip on me again. After everything I had been through, the surgeries, infections, hyperbaric treatments, navigating the complicated relationship with Dr. Z, and building The Shower Shirt Co., why was I frozen by the idea of speaking?

It made no sense. I knew my story better than anyone. I could talk through every detail, the surgery, the recovery, the challenges, and the process of bringing a product to market. And yet, the fear remained, stubborn and real.

Then it hit me. I had never fully processed the emotional trauma of the previous two years. The Shower Shirt™ had kept me busy, creating, fighting, working, and even challenging bureaucrats in Washington, D.C. But in many ways, it had also allowed me to avoid the deeper psychological impact of breast cancer on my self-worth. I had done television and print interviews and spoken about the invention, but standing in front of hundreds of people as their keynote speaker sharing my entire physical, psychological, and emotional experience for nearly an hour felt overwhelming.

This fear was different. I have never been afraid of much, aside from heights, sharks, and my father, but this was something else entirely. It was raw and intense. I kept thinking that telling my story on stage would feel like walking across the stage naked, and I did not like that idea at all. Still, I knew I had to face it.

It took me weeks to fully commit to the engagement, and even longer to begin writing the script. Putting those years into words for a one-hour talk was both cathartic and exhausting. I laughed, I cried, and I worked through more than a few boxes of tissues. It was grief, sorrow, and release all at once. Slowly, the words began to come. It felt like unpacking a heavy suitcase I had been carrying for far too long.

Then the day arrived. I walked into the room and saw 350 people, many of them breast cancer survivors. I felt everything I had feared and more, but something surprising happened. It was incredible. Sharing my story, speaking about my journey, my recovery, and the creation of The Shower Shirt™, felt liberating. The Zonta Club members were gracious, supportive, and welcoming. That first talk was phenomenal.

On the flight back to Florida, I read a quote from Nelson Mandela's autobiography, *Long Walk to Freedom*: *"After climbing a big hill, one only finds that there are so many more hills to climb."*

That stayed with me. Speaking about my journey, about what I had once described as *"walking naked across the stage,"* was a major hill. But it was not the end. It was only the beginning.

From there, the doors opened. That first engagement led to more invitations, more opportunities to share my story and speak about entrepreneurship and resilience. Each time I spoke, I learned something important. Fear may show up, but it does not get to stay. With every talk, I felt stronger, more connected, and more prepared for whatever came next.

That fall, I received another invitation that felt almost surreal. I was asked to speak at an event hosted by Walt Disney World called Go for the Greens, a business development conference for women entrepreneurs sponsored by Disney and UPS. The audience included representatives from organizations such as the National Association of Women Business Owners, the Women's Business Enterprise National Council, Women Impacting Public Policy, and the Women Presidents' Organization. It was a room full of some of the most driven women in the country.

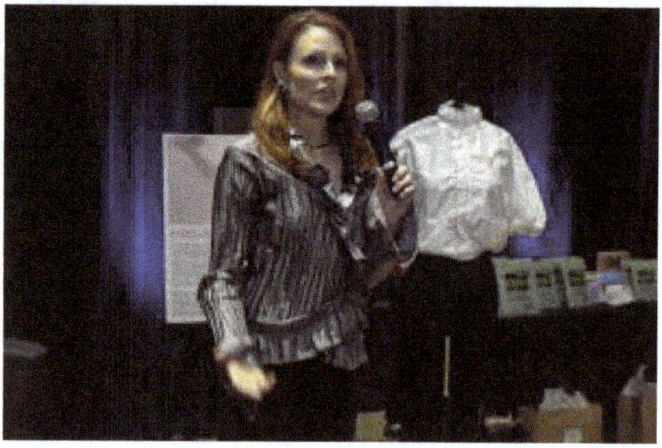

"Go for the Greens" Speaking Engagement at Walt Disney World

I was thrilled. Standing there as a keynote speaker at a breast cancer luncheon sponsored by Disney, I felt exactly where I was meant to be. By then, I had spoken at several events and no longer felt like I was walking onto the stage unprepared or exposed. The nerves had faded, replaced by excitement and purpose. I genuinely wanted to share my story in a way that could help others facing their own challenges.

From the moment I entered that room, I felt a powerful sense of connection with the women there. At first, I could not quite explain it. But after speaking with several of them, I realized what it was. They shared the same *"take the bull by the horns"* mindset I had carried my entire life.

Growing up in a male dominated household, having strong opinions was not always encouraged. But here, I was surrounded by women who were ambitious, outspoken, and relentless, just like me. The difference was that they were also lifting each other up. It was empowering to witness. That kind of support, that woman-to-woman energy, is something the world needs more of.

Looking back, it is remarkable to think that when I was diagnosed with breast cancer in 2009, giving inspirational talks was the last thing on my mind. Speaking openly about breasts, mastectomies, surgeries, infections, and hyperbaric treatments felt like something no one would want to hear. And honestly, I did not even feel ready to call my story inspirational at the time. I was still trying to understand it myself.

At 42, when my reconstructive surgeon told me I might only have one breast for the rest of my life, it was overwhelming. Those years were a rollercoaster of emotions, my first real confrontation with mortality, while also trying to understand what it meant for my health and my identity as a woman.

Even now, I am not sure anyone ever fully processes a breast cancer diagnosis. But this I do know. I have learned from it. I have grown because of it. My career trajectory changed because of it. And most importantly, it inspired me. It inspired me to become an inventor, to help other inventors, to collaborate with breast cancer support groups, to step onto stage and share my story, and ultimately, to write *Beautifully Unbroken.*

Life does not hand you the hardships you would choose, but it does give you the opportunity to turn those hardships into purpose.

CHAPTER 16

Psychological Battles of Breast Cancer

You've already heard so much about my story, the experiences I went through, the surgeries, the complications, but there's more. The parts that don't just affect your body, but rattle your mind. The real psychological battles.

As a former health and medical television reporter, and now a medical print columnist, I've interviewed hundreds of people with chronic or terminal illnesses. I've learned how to pull raw, unfiltered emotion from patients so readers can truly feel their journey. And no matter the story, my last question was always the same: *"What's the one message you want our viewers to take away?"*

Now, as I relive so much of my own breast cancer experience while writing *Beautifully Unbroken*, I ask myself that same question: *"What is it that I want my readers to take from this book?"*

Here's what I want you to know: breast cancer does not only affect physical change, but can also affect psychological change. There's life before a breast cancer diagnosis, and life after. And let me tell you, before and after are as different as black and white, night and day, Venus and Mars, which, of course, brings to mind the differences between men and women, thanks to Dr. John Gray. It's like watching the rain from inside your house versus standing in it. Inside, you stay dry. Outside, you are soaked. And after a breast cancer diagnosis, you are drenched. Soaked with fragility, sorrow, fear, and trauma.

"You have breast cancer." Those words changed my life at 41 years of age, just like they do for hundreds of thousands of women every year. That's why I want to focus on the before and after of the disease and its psychological impact.

I often wonder if my mother's death, my father's lack of paternal empathy after her passing, and my divorce a few years later all contributed to my diagnosis. Nearly a decade of chronic worry, psychological imbalance, trauma, grief, depression, and persistent anxiety created the kind of stress that can wear down the body. According to MD Anderson Cancer Center, chronic stress has a profound effect on how your body's systems function. Research shows stress does not directly cause cancer, but it can accelerate tumor growth and metastasis by weakening the immune system. Adrenaline and cortisol, the fight-or-flight hormones, can create an environment where cancer cells are more likely to thrive.

In hindsight, I believe that's what happened to me. My body was under so much emotional and psychological strain that it created the conditions for a tumor to form in my right breast and possibly set the stage for cancer in my left. Chronic fear, grief, and trying to rebuild a sense of normalcy after my mother's death and my divorce were powerful fuel.

Even now, fifteen years later, I still feel moments of FEAR, False Emotions Appearing Real, when I think about the original diagnosis, the months of treatment, the infections, and the ongoing uncertainty surrounding my reconstruction. That fear has likely added a layer of mild PTSD. According to the National Institutes of Health, that is common. Survivors often struggle with anxiety, depression, avoidance, diminished self-esteem, body image issues, and even survivor's guilt. Fatigue, sleep disturbances, and changes in identity or sexuality are also common. Add in the cognitive effects of chemotherapy, mental fog, memory lapses, and slower thinking, and it becomes clear that the psychological impact can be just as significant as the physical one.

But here's the truth: resilience is possible.

Life is about how we adapt, how we recover, and how we grow. Like a rubber band that stretches but does not break, or a tree that bends in the wind but remains rooted, resilience is not about avoiding pain. It is about developing the strength to move through it. Practices like gratitude, mindfulness, and therapy can make a meaningful difference.

It has taken me years, but I have found healthier ways to manage my emotions. When anxiety creeps in about future health complications, I talk myself through it. *"Lisa, take the emotion out of this. Focus on the facts. You are healthy today. You have no infection today. You are strong and resilient. If complications arise, you will find the best of care."* Staying grounded in reality helps me move forward.

While writing this book, I attended an Elysian Magazine Spring Wellness event in Charlotte, North Carolina, with my friend Gladys. That experience reinforced the importance of gratitude and appreciating life's even smallest blessings. During a breakout session, we were given a list of words and asked to choose the ones that resonated most. After narrowing my list, five stood out: Courage, Authenticity, Resilience, Gratitude, and Originality. Together, they formed CARGO, a personal acronym that now guides how I live my life.

On days when fear or PTSD begins to surface, I remind myself: I live by CARGO. Courage. Authenticity. Resilience. Gratitude. Originality. That framework keeps me grounded and moving forward.

As I worked through this chapter, I realized I wanted additional professional insight into the psychological impact of breast cancer. I reached out to my childhood friend, Dr. Rosezina Meadows, to collaborate. She knew my story, and through her expertise and research, we recognized that thousands of women share similar emotional experiences.

Rosezina has a remarkable ability to simplify complex emotional concepts. One principle stood out: there is life before diagnosis and life after, but in between is a profound sense of loss and bereavement. A kind of emotional death, where trust in one's body is replaced by fear.

As I close this chapter, I want to share Dr. Meadows' clinical perspective on grief in relation to breast cancer:

Grief, in simple terms, is a response to loss. And loss comes in many forms. Most people immediately think of losing a loved one, but loss can happen in countless ways: the end of a relationship, the death of a pet, losing a job, a shift in identity, illness, and certainly a breast cancer diagnosis. For anyone trying to recreate themselves after a serious illness, this process can be psychologically challenging.

Some types of grief are considered complex grief. For example, when someone loses a loved one to a terminal illness, it's common to feel both relief that the suffering is over and sadness for the loss. Similarly, if a woman requires a mastectomy due to breast cancer, she might feel relief that the cancer is gone but also deep sadness at the loss of her breast. Losing a part of one's body triggers grief that affects identity—it can disrupt your sense of purpose, values, confidence, and even your disposition and personality.

Everyone grieves differently, but some feelings are universal: shock, anger, sadness, depression, fear, and anxiety. Grief is often described in five stages: denial, anger, bargaining, depression, and acceptance. But it's important to note that grief is not linear. One day you may feel denial, the next day depression, and then swing back to anger—and that's completely normal.

Patience in grief means allowing yourself to feel intense, unpredictable emotions without any timeline or pressure to "get over it and move on." There's no right or wrong way to grieve. Patience is the strength that helps you support yourself through the process.

When dealing with grief after breast cancer specifically, it's about acknowledging and accepting, the loss of your pre-cancer life, your body image, and your sense of peace. With that acceptance, and with psychological work, you can create a healthy, mentally strong, post-cancer survival mentality. Some strategies can help navigate these emotions:

- ***Use Tools for Processing:*** *Journaling or writing down your thoughts can help validate and process complex emotions.*

- ***Seek Specialized Support:*** *Connect with others who understand, such as breast cancer support groups or oncology social workers. Organizations like CancerCare.org offer guidance for managing grief.*

- ***Validate Your Emotions:*** *Give yourself permission to feel sadness, anger, or fear without judgment. Grieving the loss of your former body, health, or sense of safety is normal.*

- ***Prioritize Self-Care:*** *Engage in activities that promote well-being, like deep breathing, meditation, gentle exercise, yoga, spending time in nature, or creative outlets such as art or music.*

- ***Manage Physical Health:*** *Attend follow-up appointments to address ongoing side effects and reduce anxiety about recurrence.*

- ***Seek Professional Help:*** *If sadness feels overwhelming or persistent, consult a therapist or psychologist, ideally one experienced with cancer survivors, for cognitive behavioral therapy (CBT) or counseling.*

- ***Utilize Healthy Supports:*** *Be open to support from family and friends. Many times, the people that love you, will feel helpless and experience vicarious grief. In other words, when you are hurting due to loss, they are hurting with you. Utilizing and allowing their support will not* *only help in your healing, but also in theirs. Remember, they are on this journey right alongside you.*

- ***Set Boundaries:*** *It's okay to limit contact with people who are not supportive, it's important to prioritize your emotional well-being.*

Grief after cancer does not follow a timeline. Patience is not about waiting for grief to end—it's about learning to live with loss. Over time, you'll find a new normal, one that allows you to thrive in a psychologically healthier way. – **Rosezina Meadows, LPCC-S, PhD.**

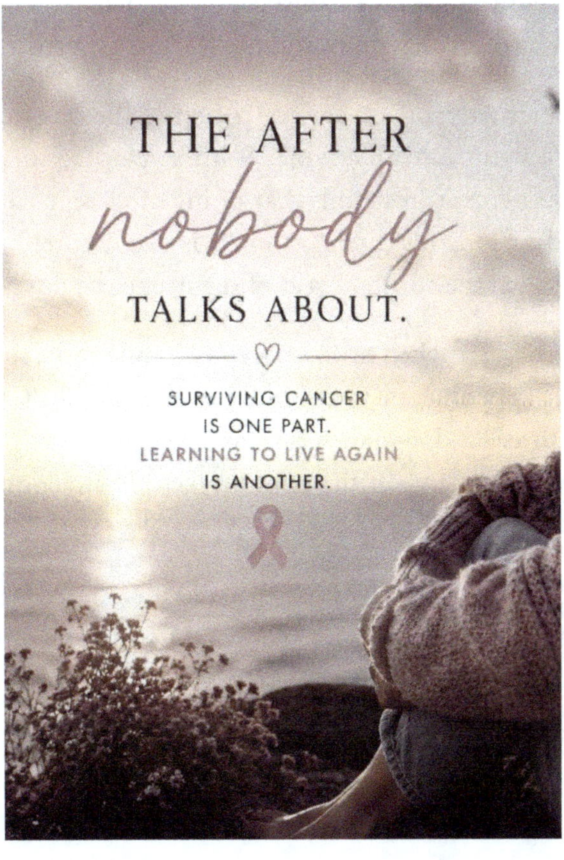

CHAPTER 17

Rocking & Reflecting

One of the most important elements of life is reflection. Reflecting on your journey, your experiences, your mistakes, your purpose, and your vision. Without reflection, it is difficult to grow. For me, it was not until after surviving breast cancer and bringing The Shower Shirt™ to market that I truly began to reflect. And yes, I have made many mistakes along the way. But I rarely make the same mistake twice. That is the value of reflection. It teaches, shapes, and moves you forward.

For many breast cancer patients, the five-year mark becomes a significant milestone. With a five-year survival rate around 90 percent, reaching that point often signals a strong likelihood of long-term remission. It is not a cure, but it is a moment when the constant fear of recurrence begins to ease.

When I reached my own five-year milestone, something else was happening in parallel. The Shower Shirt Co. had reached three and a half years as the only water-resistant mastectomy garment on the U.S. market. That alignment felt deeply personal and professional.

Around that time, a friend asked me, *"So, is The Shower Shirt Co. rocking and rolling yet?"* I paused before answering. Then I said, *"It's rocking."*

And it was.

Thousands of shirts had been sold across the United States and internationally. Retailers, hospital systems, and online platforms were carrying the product. We had strong patent protection and growing brand recognition. But I could not say we were truly "rolling" until we secured Medicare coverage or meaningful legislative progress.

Eventually, it became clear there was not enough bipartisan support to move the Post-Mastectomy Infection Reduction Act forward. Some lawmakers cited cost concerns. And yes, reimbursement costs money. But preventing post-surgical infections is far less expensive than treating them. At a retail price of $78, the product remained accessible as a self-pay option.

At that point, I had to accept a difficult truth. Even if I had dedicated myself fully to the legislation, it likely would not have passed without significant lobbying resources, tens of thousands of dollars per month, with no guarantee of success. And that was okay. I had done everything I could.

What mattered was what I learned. I had engaged with policymakers, educated decision-makers, and brought attention to a real gap in patient care. Most importantly, the product existed. Women finally had a solution that provided protection and dignity.

The Shower Shirt Co. also reached a major milestone. We became debt-free.

From the beginning, inventory and patent costs were our biggest financial hurdles. I initially funded the company myself, but after our first 500 units sold, the business began to sustain itself. With the patience of partners like our attorney and manufacturing team, we were able to pay down every balance. That moment brought a sense of relief I will never forget.

At the same time, my professional life shifted. The healthcare system I worked for was acquired by a national for-profit organization. While the transition created uncertainty, it ultimately became an opportunity. Within ten days, I secured four media consulting contracts with local physicians. I was earning more and had greater flexibility than ever before.

That flexibility changed everything. It allowed me to invest more time in growing the business. I paid off two of my three mortgages and gained a level of financial stability that brought real peace of mind.

With that stability came growth. We expanded for additional plus sizing through our manufacturing partner, producing smaller runs and bringing new options to market much faster than before.

Reaching the five-year survivorship mark brought a different kind of clarity. The previous years had been filled with constant change, physically, emotionally, and professionally. But now, for the first time, I could see a sense of calm ahead.

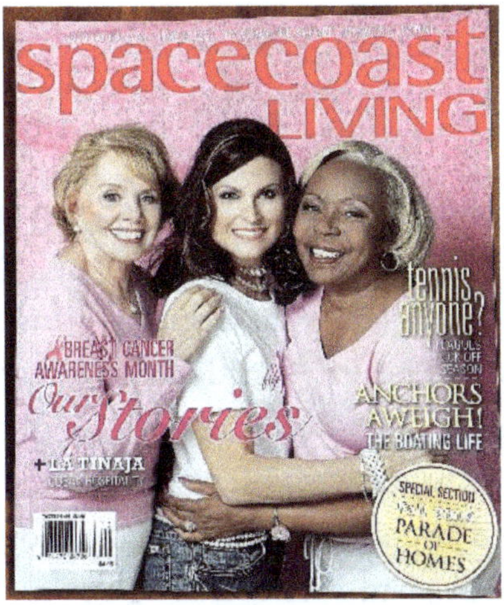

Space Coast Living, 2014

I took a deep breath, said a prayer, and prepared for whatever came next.

For the first time in a long time, everything felt aligned.

And looking back, I realized I had found a rhythm: rocking, rolling, and reflecting.

CHAPTER 18

Oh No, Not Again!

For nearly ten years after my breast cancer diagnosis, I had been overall healthy. Aside from a few broken bones and lingering nasal infections linked to the original MRSA infection, I managed well. I stayed proactive about my immune system. I paid attention. I did not take shortcuts. I understood that my body had been through war, and I treated it accordingly.

By then, The Shower Shirt Co. was doing well. What had once been an idea born from necessity had grown into a steady, respected product helping patients around the world. Around the same time, I found myself leaning more toward writing guest columns on alternative and homeopathic wellness solutions than toward evidence-based medical features. I was ghostwriting for physicians, helping them shape their clinical expertise into words non-clinical readers could understand. It felt purposeful. It felt stable. Life, for once, felt like it was not constantly slipping through my hands.

I let myself believe I was finally on the other side of it all. But then came 2020.

As it did for so many, the year brought loss. My Aunt Faye passed away. We never received clear answers about the cause, but the timing pointed to COVID, quietly making its way into our communities before anyone fully grasped what was coming. The uncertainty was its own kind of pain. There was no clear place to put the grief, no explanation to hold onto. It just sat there, heavy, and unresolved.

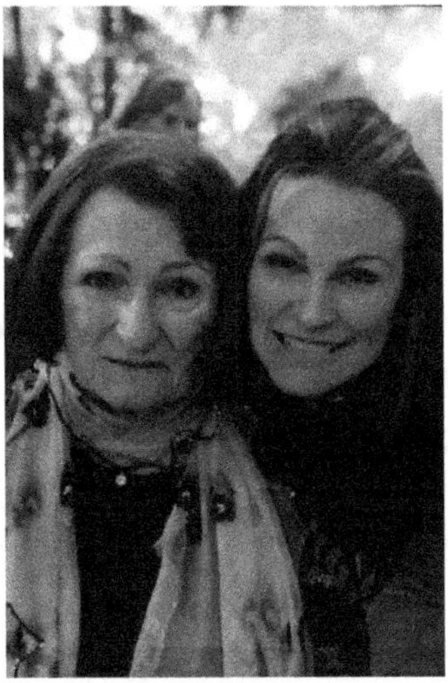

Me and my Aunt Faye

That fall, I began to feel different. Not dramatically ill, just off. It was not sudden. There was no moment I could point to and say, this is when it started. It was slower than that, almost easy to dismiss at first. But I felt a contrast, not like myself. Stress hit me differently. Things that I used to manage without thinking now felt overwhelming. My patience wore thin in ways that did not feel like me.

And then there was something I could not ignore.

Every now and then, my head would tremble. Just slightly. Small enough that someone else might not notice, but I did. I always did. And each time it happened, something inside me tightened.

One day, I asked my husband, *"Is my head shaking?"* He looked at me and said, *"It looks like your hair is shaking a small amount."*

We were deep in the COVID era by then. The world was anxious. My father was ill again. I was studying for my MBA. We were navigating isolation, fear, nonstop news, and the strange stillness of lockdowns. I assumed it was stress. Too much caffeine. Too much on my mind, a perfect storm. I brushed it aside.

A few months later, in March 2021, I was rushed by ambulance to the emergency department with severe abdominal pain. The diagnosis came quickly and bluntly: cecal volvulus. A rare, life-threatening emergency caused by the twisting of the colon, leading to intestinal obstruction.

The surgeon explained that if I did not go into surgery immediately, my colon could burst. Sepsis could set in. I could die.

Breast cancer had given me time to think. Time to research. Time to consider options and second opinions. This was different. I was sitting in the emergency room, being told there was no choice. Surgery was happening now.

I like choices. I like knowledge before decisions. Knowledge is power. I like to feel some sense of control. On March 3, 2021, I had none.

When I woke up, I had been cut open, nearly hip to hip, with a long road of recovery ahead. Healing from emergency abdominal surgery is physically painful, yes, but also mentally disorienting. It is abrupt. It does not allow emotional preparation. You go from functioning to vulnerable in a matter of hours. I had been at the Cocoa Beach Health & Fitness that morning doing a "butts and guts" class. That evening, I lay in a hospital bed with an eight-inch incision.

The unofficial diagnosis for the twisting of my colon was years of colonics, procedures that flush the large intestine with water for detoxification and improved digestion. My surgeon said my colon was stretched, more like that of a 75-year-old than a 55-year-old. I accepted his theory, given my history of detoxifying disciplines.

As I was recovering over the next two months, another kind of trauma unfolded. It was not medical, but it cut just as deeply.

In May 2021, I learned that the widow of one of my husband's friends had begun pursuing him just two months after her husband passed away. At first, it sounded almost unbelievable. Then it became impossible to ignore. Her behavior was aggressive and relentless. When she did not get the response she wanted, it escalated into threats. What started as unsettling quickly became something much more serious. It felt chaotic. It felt intrusive. It felt alarming.

He told her to leave him alone. In response, she threatened to harm herself, jumping from a balcony, and overdosing on prescription medication. He often referenced the film *Fatal Attraction*, worried we might come home to something equally theatrical and disturbing.

The stress from that situation was relentless. Not loud every day, but constant. My nervous system never fully relaxed. Around that time, my cranium began to hurt in a way I had never experienced, needles pressing into my scalp, sharp, repetitive, deep, day in and day out for weeks. I did not know it then, but I was beginning to have multiple minor strokes.

A few weeks later, I sat in a neurologist's office, uneasy, waiting to review the results of a brain MRI. I was unprepared for what I was about to hear.

The neurologist told me the scan showed frontal lobe atrophy and cerebellum atrophy. The cerebellum damage, he explained, was causing essential tremors in my head. He also said I had experienced five minor strokes.

I asked if they were TIAs, strokes that cause temporary symptoms without lasting damage. He said no. TIAs do not leave scar tissue. My MRI showed scarring.

Shock washed over me, the kind that makes the room feel distant, as if I am watching myself receive the news from across the table. Frontal lobe. Cerebellum. Atrophy. Scar tissue.

Then he asked a question I did not expect: was I a drug addict or an alcoholic? He explained that my brain scan, at 55, resembled that of a 75 year-old.

I looked at him calmly. *"Doctor Packey, this is one of the cleanest bodies you will ever find."*

Even in shock, I could not ignore the coincidence: for the second time in nine months, a doctor had told me a part of my body had progressed two decades older than my age. In that moment, I thought my life as I knew it was over. I imagined living the rest of my years with extreme head tremors. I imagined cognitive decline accelerating. My brain throbbed constantly, felt inflamed, geriatric, twenty years ahead of schedule.

I had to confront the possibility that I might never be the same, that I might never work again, or live as an active, mid-fifties woman. That thought alone was shocking.

The months that followed were disorienting. I could not remember simple things. My mind felt wrapped in fog. I would search for basic words mid-sentence. Forget names, dates. Lose track of days. Be emotional, impulsive, and inconsistent in problem-solving. Forget how to spell simple words. These were all effects of frontal lobe atrophy and brain injury from strokes.

I was trying to run a company. Meet journalism deadlines. Yet on some days, I could barely organize my thoughts long enough to answer an email.

For six months, my neurologist adjusted medications carefully to reduce tremors without adding cognitive side effects. Amid it all, he gave me one instruction that surprised me: keep writing. He said it would be good for my brain, cognitively and neurologically. Challenge it, he said, do not retreat.

So I wrote. Even on days when it felt like pushing through mud. Even in severe pain. Even when I could barely converse.

I considered retiring. I called a disability attorney to explore my options. He said I would likely qualify for disability.

Emotionally, though, that didn't feel authentic. Giving up would have felt like defeat. I was used to taking the difficult road.

Once I removed emotion from the decision, I realized my soul, determination, and tenacity were stronger than any neurological diagnosis.

I began researching brain atrophy. Common causes appeared first: drug abuse, alcoholism, which explained the neurologist's question. I also found research linking brain atrophy to ischemia (interrupted oxygen to the brain), triggering strokes, chronic anxiety, depression, migraines, certain medications, and even repeated anesthesia. Multiple surgeries over the years compounded the effect. It was cumulative, not a single event.

Looking back, I am still amazed at the human psyche. Instead of surrendering, I became determined to support my brain. I meditated several times a week. Added daily yoga and intense cardio to boost circulation. Reduced inflammation through diet: more fruits and vegetables, healthy fats, cutting carbs, and refined sugar. Incorporated anti-inflammatory spices like turmeric and garlic.

I studied herbal medicine, Ayurvedic practices, and nutrition for cognitive health. I incorporated supplements like neurotropic and nootropic blends, mushroom extracts, ginkgo biloba, ginseng, bacopa, ashwagandha, and cocoa flavanols. A friend, Dr. Christina, created a zeolite-based detox product that I added daily. Evenings included a red-light therapy hat to increase circulation.

I continued evidence-based medical care, appointments, medications, and monitoring progress.

Emotionally and spiritually, I had work to do, too. I had to process anger towards my husband for not disclosing what had happened. However, I understood his fear and intent to shield me while I recovered from another medical misfortune. That forgiveness required much conversation, accountability, and time. But a requirement for spiritual healing to release the anger.

Nearly five years have passed since that MRI. Through medical management, lifestyle improvements, ongoing cognitive exercises, and persistence, my neurological deficits are also now managed. I remain mindful, monitor stress, support my brain with herbal remedies, and strengthen disrupted neural pathways through repetition and patience. Some functions operate differently, and I accept that.

The moral of this chapter? Yes, discernment and boundaries are critical. But the deeper lesson is grit. Mental stamina. Refusing to let a medical diagnosis, a marital learning experience, or a brain MRI define your life, or the end of your story.

CHAPTER 19
The Perfect Exit

When I look back over the decades, what stands out most is not the successes or the setbacks, but the steady thread of resilience that carried me through both. My life did not unfold in a straight line. It curved, stalled, accelerated, and at times felt as though it completely unraveled. Yet somehow, each season prepared me for the next.

I was raised in a home that was both loving and structured. In many ways, my early life was sheltered and privileged. We worked hard, but we were also given opportunities that many families around us did not have or simply could not afford. While some of my girlfriends were unable to take piano lessons, dance classes, or gymnastics training, I participated in all three. At the time, I did not see it as privilege. It was simply my normal.

It was not until college that I began to understand how fortunate I had been. I realized that not every parent could or would pay for their child's education. That awareness shifted something in me. My parents had not only provided me with opportunities but had instilled a deep sense of gratitude. They taught me stewardship: to appreciate what we had and use it wisely. That mindset has stayed with me throughout my life.

Outside that sheltered beginning, however, life was not gentle.

After college, breaking into the news industry felt nearly impossible. I had always wanted to cover health and medical stories and believed I could do it well. But belief does not open doors. I faced rejection after rejection. I questioned my abilities. I wondered if I had misjudged my calling.

During those same years, my personal life was unstable. I moved through several unhealthy relationships, each teaching me lessons I had not wanted to learn. Around that time, I was also diagnosed with premenstrual dysphoric disorder. For two weeks each month, I battled severe migraines, a possible contributor to my eventual brain atrophy. Managing a full-time role in health and medical news while navigating these emotional lows required a level of discipline I had not anticipated. Luckily, the female body tends to evolve hormonally over time, and that diagnosis resolved itself after a few years.

Television added another layer. Being on camera meant that confidence mattered. Appearance mattered. Composure mattered. I was no longer simply writing stories; I was delivering them visibly and publicly. I felt as though I was constantly proving myself, both professionally and personally.

My twenties were far more difficult than I expected. They stripped away naivety and replaced it with experience. In many ways, those years prepared me for my thirties, which brought even greater trials. My mother's death changed me in ways I still cannot fully articulate. A divorce forced me to reevaluate my understanding of commitment and identity. A breast cancer diagnosis confronted me with mortality.

Through each decade, I survived. I learned. I adapted. The lessons of my twenties informed my thirties. The trials of my thirties strengthened my forties. My fifties demanded yet another level of resilience. As I approach my sixties, I see the progression clearly and, fortunately, I feel mentally stronger than ever. As the saying goes, *"What does not break you builds you."*

My girlfriends and I used to talk about what we wanted in our twenties, careers, relationships, building a life that looked successful. By our thirties, priorities shifted. By our forties and fifties, they shifted again. Stability mattered more. Health mattered more. Peace mattered more.

For me, the last thirty years have been about building: a career, a real estate portfolio, a company, a life after loss. Apart from my divorce twenty years ago, I rarely considered exits. I was oriented towards endurance.

Exits, however, are part of life, jobs, relationships, seasons, and even businesses.

A few months ago, I was introduced to Robert Green, author of *The Better Exit*. The book outlines the importance of having an exit plan, particularly in business. The concept is practical and straightforward: build intentionally, but also prepare thoughtfully for transition. His ideas resonated with me more than I expected.

For years, two of my business mentors, Beth Gitlin and Jeanette Kraar, reminded me, *"Lisa, you need an exit plan for The Shower Shirt Co."* My response was always the same: *"I created this company to help breast cancer patients shower after mastectomy surgery. I did not invent it for financial gain."*

That was true. The product was born out of my own diagnosis. It was cathartic. It gave meaning to a painful season. My vision for the company was emotional and philanthropic, not corporate. I focused on service, not strategy.

Because of that, I resisted conversations about selling or succession. An exit plan felt transactional, almost cold. I did not want to reduce something so personal to a spreadsheet.

Until recently, when something changed.

One day, I realized I was ready to sell. I was ready to focus on my next chapter.

The Shower Shirt™ had felt like my child. I gave it life. Nurtured it through early challenges. Guided it through manufacturing, distribution, and market education. Protected it. But eventually, I began to see that it might need someone else, a larger organization to take it further, someone with a different skill set, eager to scale it in ways I had never prioritized.

In my mind, I had raised it through high school. Perhaps it was time for another steward to guide it through college and beyond.

That realization led to an uncomfortable question: What is my plan?

For the first time, I understood the wisdom behind the advice I had dismissed. According to *The Better Exit*, citing the Business Enterprise Institute, at least 66% of businesses in this country do not have a written transition plan. Owners are consumed with daily operations, growth, and financial performance. Selling is rarely considered until they are emotionally ready. I was no different.

I had been so focused on running the company, living life, and overseeing journalism priorities that I had never outlined a clear strategy for stepping away. When the moment came, I felt both clarity and unpreparedness.

This decision has taught me that stewardship is not only about building and protecting, it is also about knowing when to release. An exit does not mean failure. It can represent maturity, foresight, and trust that what you created can thrive beyond you.

For someone who once avoided exits, I am learning that they are not endings. They are transitions. Sometimes, they are the most responsible step forward. So, let me tell you how teachings from *The Better Exit* evolved into "my perfect exit."

Once I allowed myself to think strategically, the next steps unfolded more smoothly than anticipated. After several meetings with a business broker, we officially listed The Shower Shirt Co., LLC for sale. It felt surreal to see it positioned that way, described in valuation terms rather than personal history.

Within a few months, after 14 years of building, refining, and protecting it, the company was acquired.

The transition was professional and respectful. No dramatic crescendo, no grand farewell. Just paperwork, negotiations, signatures, and the quiet realization that something significant had shifted. What I had once cradled as an idea during one of the hardest seasons of my life now belonged to someone else.

The moral of this part of the story is clear: whether your planned exit is two years away or twenty, implementing solid exit principles strengthens a business. It forces clarity. It builds value. It makes the company more stable and more transferable. Even if you never sell, operating with that discipline creates a healthier enterprise.

As one major chapter closed, another opened almost immediately.

Within days of starting sales negotiations, a publishing house approached me about writing this autobiography, *Beautifully Unbroken*. The premise: to chronicle my journey and the lessons drawn from it.

My first response was immediate and firm: *"No! I am not interested. And why would anyone want to read my story?"*

It was the same reaction I had years earlier when invited to speak publicly. Who am I to stand in front of a room? Who am I to author a book?

The publishers were persistent. They created a detailed outline based on past media features, speaking engagements, and milestones. When I read it, I was unexpectedly emotional. Seeing the events laid out, the losses, recoveries, risks, and rebuilding, moved me to tears. I told them I would think about it.

I shared the outline with trusted friends in media and publishing. The response was consistent: *"Go for it!"*

One of those individuals was a former colleague, and friend, Bob Stover, an executive newspaper editor for decades who said, *"Lisa, the book outline is remarkable. I encourage you to proceed with this opportunity. It is inspirational, has a high ceiling, and I believe will resonate with many audiences."*

One of my closest friends, whom I affectionately call *"the best little sister in the world,"* Kim Mooty, said something that stayed with me: *"Lisa, this is a gift from God. You do not turn a gift from God down."* Her words settled into my spirit.

Besides trusted friends, I agreed to move forward for one primary reason, the same reason I invented The Shower Shirt™: if this book can help even one person, it will be worth it.

If it helps one cancer patient feel less alone. One breast cancer survivor, who is exhausted and discouraged. One inventor, doubting that a painful idea could become meaningful. One woman who has lost her mother. One person seeking entrepreneurship. One Christian struggling with doubt. One person, more spiritual than religious, but seeking something deeper.

If it reaches even one heart, every vulnerable page will be worth writing.

And now, some news that breaks my heart. While working on this book, my father passed away. We laid him to rest on December 27th, just two days after Christmas. I was sailing through Asia, on a Princess Cruise, immersed in this manuscript, when the call came. The world, yet again, felt smaller, colder, and infinitely heavier. Grief does not schedule itself conveniently.

One of the last conversations I had with him occurred two months before he died. I said, *"Daddy, can you believe it? I have a book deal. A few years ago, I thought my life was over when I was diagnosed with brain atrophy and learned I had neurological tremors and strokes. And now, publishers are asking me to write an autobiography. Can you believe it?"*

In his familiar John Wayne southern drawl, delivered with an Archie Bunker disposition, he replied, *"Lisa, once those publishers learn you are the daughter of a Midwest farmer who wears overalls, they just might pull that book deal."*

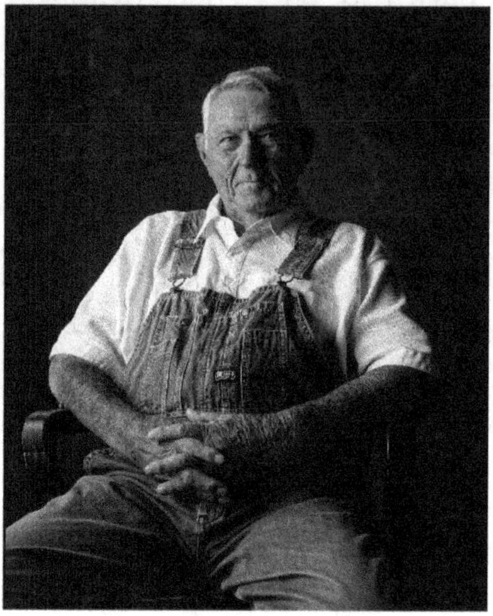

GARY CRITES

(May 8, 1939, to December 6, 2025)
Credit: Joe Craig, The Missouri Farm Project

I laughed. That was my father: grounded, humble, never overly impressed. His humor steadied me, even in that moment.

Soon after, I read a quote by Katherine Whitehorn, a British journalist and author: *"One reason we are so stricken when our parents die is that the audience you've been aiming at all your life, shocking it, pleasing it, has suddenly left the theatre."* So true. I feel those words even more now that both my parents are gone.

Looking back, God's timing was impeccable, yet again. Selling The Shower Shirt Co. did not just provide what Robert Green would call a better exit, it felt like the perfect exit. It freed space. Created margin. Allowed me to step into another therapeutic venture.

Authoring this book has been healing. It required revisiting carefully packed-away trauma. It demanded honesty about fear, doubt, and weakness. There were days when laughter through tears was the only appropriate response. Nights when I questioned whether I could tell the story or even finish it. On those days, I prayed for guidance and strength to complete this project, this 'gift' of opportunity, as my friend called it.

And once again, I was carried through fear, through false emotions, through hesitation, into obedience. God carried me through this book, just as He carried me through my mother's death, and the creation of The Shower Shirt™. He has always carried me when I needed Him.

Becoming a published author or an inventor was never on my childhood list of ambitions. Yet here I am, beyond blessed.

My hope is that *Beautifully Unbroken* supports you as you read it, just as writing it supported me. Stories connect us across circumstances. They remind us that resilience is possible, even when it feels distant.

A portion of the proceeds from each book will be shared with nonprofit organizations and breast cancer support groups. A mission that began more than fifteen years ago, when I simply wanted to help women shower safely after mastectomy surgery, continues in another form. The same patient population that inspired The Shower Shirt™ will benefit again, this time through words instead of fabric.

In the end, that continuity feels right. What began as survival evolved into service. What felt like an ending became a transition. And what once appeared broken has, in many ways, become *"beautifully unbroken."*

"Healing doesn't mean the damage never existed. It means the damage no longer controls your life. – Akshay Dubey (Author of the Success Journey)

www.ingramcontent.com/pod-product-compliance
Lightning Source LLC
LaVergne TN
LVHW022023051126
851858LV00003B/21
* 9 7 8 1 9 9 7 0 4 0 2 9 3 *